Praise for D

"I had always thought that there was little one could do to prevent or slow the symptoms of Alzheimer's. However, in this amazing book, *Defeating Dementia*, Dr. Richard Furman explains in an easy to understand and detailed way that there are actually things you can be doing right now to decrease your odds of developing Alzheimer's dementia. This book can change the way you live. It can give you a new hope and practical steps to deal with—and even help prevent—Alzheimer's."

Franklin Graham, president and CEO
of the Billy Graham Evangelistic Association
and founder of Samaritan's Purse, from the foreword

"While many books have been written about individuals with Alzheimer's, none has so seamlessly connected the disease biology, the patient experience, and the preventative science as Dr. Furman does so skillfully. Dr. Furman's work will serve as the definitive guide on preventative measures to decrease one's chances of developing Alzheimer's dementia."

Senator Bill Frist, nationally recognized heart and lung
transplant surgeon, former US Senate majority leader,
and chairman of the executive council
of Cressey and Company, from the foreword

"Dr. Furman has created a unique book for the public—one that synthesizes decades of research on the prevention and early treatment of dementia into understandable chunks and practical advice. Pairing the science with personal story provides immediacy, underscoring that this advice is not just a good idea, it's crucial and matters now."

Dr. Richard Ackermann, director, Hospice & Palliative
Medicine Fellowship, Mercer University School of Medicine;
Hospice physician of Mrs. Dell

Praise for *Your Cholesterol Matters*

"A wealth of knowledge for everyone interested in improving their health. Excellent guidelines with clear understanding."

Tim Edmisten, MD, FACS, past president,
North Carolina American College of Surgeons

Praise for *Prescription for Life*

"Dr. Furman lays out a thorough review of the medical literature, written in layman's terms in such a way that is easily understood. Read it. Apply it. If you are like the majority of Americans, you will become 7–12 years younger physiologically than you presently are chronologically."

Bill Frist, nationally recognized heart and lung transplant surgeon, former US Senate majority leader, and chairman of the executive council of Cressey and Company

"While many respond negatively to the thought of exercising, dieting, and changing their lifestyle, Dr. Furman has managed to take what is threatening and make it thrilling. When you finish this read, you will actually be excited about the possibility of a longer, healthier life."

Dr. David Jeremiah, from the foreword

WINNING YOUR
BLOOD SUGAR
BATTLE

How to Prevent and
Control Type 2 Diabetes

RICHARD FURMAN, MD, FACS

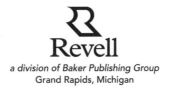
Revell
a division of Baker Publishing Group
Grand Rapids, Michigan

Published by Revell
a division of Baker Publishing Group
PO Box 6287, Grand Rapids, MI 49516-6287
www.revellbooks.com

Printed in the United States of America

Library of Congress Cataloging-in-Publication Data
Names: Furman, Richard, author.
Title: Winning your blood sugar battle : how to prevent and control Type 2 diabetes
   / Richard Furman, MD, FACS.
Description: Grand Rapids, MI : Revell, a division of Baker Publishing Group,
   [2019]
Identifiers: LCCN 2018045118 | ISBN 9780800728069 (pbk.)
Subjects: LCSH: Non-insulin-dependent diabetes—Popular works. | Non-insulin-
   dependent diabetes—Prevention. | Non-insulin-dependent diabetes—Treatment.
   | Lifestyles.
Classification: LCC RC662.18 .F86 2019 | DDC 616.4/624—dc23
LC record available at https://lccn.loc.gov/2018045118

Some names and details have been changed to protect the privacy of the individuals involved.

This publication is intended to provide helpful and informative material on the subjects addressed. Readers should consult their personal health professionals before adopting any of the suggestions in this book or drawing inferences from it. The author and publisher expressly disclaim responsibility for any adverse effects arising from the use or application of the information contained in this book.

The author is represented by the literary agency of Wolgemuth & Associates, Inc.

19 20 21 22 23 24 25   7 6 5 4 3 2 1

In keeping with biblical principles of creation stewardship, Baker Publishing Group advocates the responsible use of our natural resources. As a member of the Green Press Initiative, our company uses recycled paper when possible. The text paper of this book is composed in part of post-consumer waste.

To my sweet wife, Harriet.

There are many virtuous and capable women in the world,
but you surpass them all!

PROVERBS 31:29 (NLT)

Contents

Introduction

The woman looked distraught as she approached me, and I could detect a tear forming at the edge of each eye. I waited for her to speak.

She slipped a tissue out of her pocket and lightly dabbed her eyes. "I just saw my doctor, and he told me I have diabetes. Type 2."

I looked at her without showing emotion. She was a nurse, and I didn't think being told she had diabetes was enough to make her cry. But then she broke down and let the tears flow.

"The bad part," she said, "the part I don't understand, is that he said being told I have diabetes is just like being told I've had my first heart attack."

Now I understood why she was so emotional. Being told she had diabetes was bad enough. Learning it was the equivalent of having a heart attack was almost more than she could take.

"I'm not sure where to begin doing something about it," she said. "I'm a nurse, but I've never really studied diabetes. I've seen a lot of the results of heart attacks, though."

She had no idea what relationship diabetes had to the health of her heart, but I knew what she was up against. I also knew she could make lifestyle changes to reduce the medication she would have to take, or even to get her off medication completely.

The complications from diabetes are the seventh leading cause of death in America, yet this book is about hope. Combating diabetes takes much more than medicine, and with lifestyle changes, you can not only treat diabetes; you can prevent it.

Let's take this journey together.

PART 1

⟶

UNDERSTANDING DIABETES

1. The Diabetes Problem

The 2017 National Diabetes Statistics Report states that 30.3 million adults in the United States have been diagnosed with diabetes. That's over 12 percent of all adults, and most of them were no doubt surprised to learn they had it.

Approximately 84 million American adults have what's called prediabetes, which means their blood sugar is above the normal range but not high enough to be medically diagnosed as diabetes. Yet 90 percent of them don't know they have it.

Either way, one out of three adults has something going on in their body that can lead to an extremely serious disease.

Both prediabetes and diabetes place you at a greater risk of having heart attacks and strokes. The information about prediabetes in this book applies to diabetes because the ongoing process in your body is the same with both. Advancing from being prediabetic to diabetic is the same process as progressing further with diabetes. So study the reports concerning prediabetes as intensely as you study the ones that cover diabetes. It's all the same disease, just in different degrees.

The more you know from a medical standpoint, the easier it will be for you to change your lifestyle. Once you realize what certain foods lead to, you'll want to change your eating habits to avoid them. Once you know the statistics concerning the effectiveness of exercise in defeating diabetes, you'll want to get off that couch. And when you see the reports concerning excess weight, you'll want to change what you eat now so you can lose that excess weight by eating foods that fill you up, yet have the fewest calories.

This book reviews the best medical research available on diabetes. As you read it, you'll realize that if you don't attack the issues with your blood sugar, you'll physiologically grow older than your chronological age. Not only will your years be difficult as you age, but you'll shorten your life span. The more you know medically, the more motivation you'll have to change your focus from treating only your blood sugar numbers to beating the problems that go hand in hand with being diabetic.

Types of Diabetes

The three types of diabetes are gestational, type 1, and type 2.

Gestational diabetes develops in pregnant women who have never had diabetes before but have developed an elevated blood glucose level during pregnancy. It affects up to 9 percent of pregnant women. It usually resolves after childbirth, but it increases the risk of developing type 2 diabetes after pregnancy. Such patients are screened and followed.

Type 1 is often hereditary, unpreventable, and shows up many times in children and young adults. Only about 5 percent of all diabetics have type 1. In type 1 the immune system attacks the islet cells in the pancreas that produce insulin. Once those cells are destroyed, the pancreas doesn't make insulin. The individual with a type 1 diagnosis will need to be given insulin.

Type 2 diabetics have the islet cells in their pancreas, but cells that receive glucose build up so much resistance to the insulin that the pancreas is called on to produce an extra amount to try to get the glucose out of the bloodstream and into the resistant cells. I picture this process as a key that has trouble fitting into a stubborn lock. After a while, the islet cells can't produce enough insulin to overcome the faulty, swollen locks in the doors of the receiver body cells to get the glucose out of the blood and into the cells. When the process first begins, where the body cells are building up a resistance against the insulin, there may be no symptoms. That's why the individual doesn't realize they're in the process of becoming diabetic.

Type 2 diabetes frequently results from being overweight and sedentary and eating improperly. The question is, Where do you begin the battle? As I indicated before, whether you're prediabetic or fully diabetic, you can definitely have hope for the prevention or reversal of the disease.

There is a marked difference between treating and curing diabetes. Most people told they have diabetes immediately begin thinking about what medicine they're going to have to take the rest of their lives. Instead they should be thinking about lifestyle changes that might reverse the diagnosis or at least reduce the medication they will have to take otherwise. Diabetes is curable, but not with medication.

The only possibility for real cure comes through eating properly, exercising, and reaching your ideal weight. This book focuses on the details of developing the proper lifestyle to fight diabetes with all your might.

How Your Body Processes Sugar

Everyone knows if you have diabetes you have a problem with how your body handles sugar. How does that process work? The nutrient that energizes the cells in our bodies is glucose. Most of our foods are broken down into glucose, which is transported through the blood. Both fat and protein will eventually be broken down into glucose. Glucose is the driving force for our energy. Our cells need glucose for energy, but the door to each cell doesn't remain open for glucose to simply float into that cell whenever it's needed.

I like to think of the process as if there were a small lock on the door of each cell and a key is necessary to unlock that door to allow the glucose to enter. Our body has a way of keeping track of how much glucose is floating around in the blood, and when it increases, a sensor goes off in our pancreas, which begins to secrete insulin. Think of insulin as that key working its way into that lock on the door of a cell to unlock it and let some glucose inside.

Most people think diabetes is caused by too much sugar in the blood, which forces the pancreas to produce more insulin than it normally should. That's half right. I'm reminded of a sign I saw in front of a little country church. It read, "Remember: a half-truth is still a whole lie." It's true that diabetes means you have too much glucose in your blood, which then requires your body to produce more than the normal amount of insulin to try to get the glucose into your cells for nutrition. But that's only half the truth.

The other side of the equation is the *why* question. Why does your body need more than the normal amount of insulin to get the sugar into the cells? If X amount of glucose is in the blood, then the switch in your body tells the pancreas to produce X amount of insulin, which is the exact amount it takes to get the X amount of glucose into the cells. But with diabetes, sugar can't enter the cells as easily as it should. That leaves excess sugar in the bloodstream, and that extra amount signals the pancreas to produce even more insulin. The initial problem is not extra glucose, but that the glucose is having difficulty getting into the cells. Something is causing that keyhole to swell, which prevents the insulin key from working properly.

As the process advances from prediabetes to full-blown diabetes, the pancreas can't keep up with the amount of insulin the body is telling it to produce, and medication must be given to control the excess glucose.

Understanding Your Blood Sugar Levels

A blood test checking your blood sugar level is important, because you and your doctor need to know some basic numbers to evaluate your condition. A normal fasting glucose is below 100mg per deciliter. Prediabetes is from 100 to 125mg; diabetes is 126 and above. Fasting glucose tests are done after a fast of eight hours. An oral glucose tolerance test is when you're given a particular sweetened drink and your glucose is tested two hours later. A diagnosis of diabetes is made if your results are 200 mg/dl or higher.

The hemoglobin A1c test measures average glucose levels over a two- to three-month period. The A1c measures what percentage of your hemoglobin—a protein in your red blood cells that carries oxygen—is coated with sugar. The worse your glucose control is, the more sugar is coated on the hemoglobin. Diabetes is diagnosed at an A1c of 6.5 percent or greater. Someone who has just been diagnosed as diabetic will likely realize they had prediabetes long before they had diabetes. As I mentioned before, most people who develop type 2 diabetes have had what is called "prediabetes," where the glucose level is above normal but not to the diabetic diagnostic number.

If someone realizes they're prediabetic, they can begin lifestyle changes that most likely will prevent their reaching a diabetic diagnosis. The problem is *prediabetes has no clear symptoms*, so most prediabetics have no idea something bad is going on in their body.

The information you're about to read applies to both the prediabetic and the diabetic, because the disease is a progression from being able to normally control your blood sugar all the way to extreme associated problems.

2. Understanding Diabetes

When most patients are told they have diabetes, their physicians briefly discuss lifestyle changes they need to make and then write a prescription for medication to help get their blood glucose down to within a normal range. Most patients take the medicine, follow up on their glucose levels, and then feel satisfied that they're "controlling" their sugar. I asked a diabetes specialist why the lifestyle changes aren't discussed in more detail with new diabetic patients. His response was to the point.

He explained that, first, most diabetic patients simply will not commit to changing their habits to take care of their glucose problem. If a doctor gives them medication, that's good enough for them. Most are overweight and don't exercise. They don't have the necessary desire to lose weight or exercise or change their diet.

Second, neither he nor any other doctor has the time to detail for each patient how they can change their lifestyle. It takes time to explain what diet to follow and why exercise is so necessary to reach their ideal weight.

Those were the two reasons the physician gave me for why

19

diabetics primarily rely on medication rather than lifestyle changes. I wondered, *What if a physician did take time to explain these things?* That's why I wrote this book. The lifestyle changes you can make will help you gain control not only of your glucose level, but also of your overall health. Your physician may not have the time to coach you, but this book will get you started on the right path.

Let's take the first explanation—that individuals simply will not commit to doing what it takes to make changes to their lifestyle.

I understand that most diabetic patients think it's simpler to just take medicine. That's probably how I would respond in such a situation. But if your doctor had the time to explain what's taking place in your body and outline precise lifestyle changes that both address blood sugar levels and help you avoid multiple health problems down the road, you would look at the situation differently.

I believe the more someone understands what's going on medically, the more likely they'll do what it takes to protect their health. The more knowledge and the more understanding they have about what's going on in their body when they have diabetes, the more likely they are to begin making changes that can make a difference.

That's exactly what happened to me one day when I read a medical article that encouraged me to consider changing my diet to prevent a medical problem.

My Revelation

That morning I had operated on a patient with blockage buildup in his left carotid artery, which had resulted in a stroke. He had been referred to me so I could remove the blockage and prevent further strokes. His carotid artery was 95 percent blocked and needed to be cleaned out.

I felt so proud of the success of the procedure. I had made a two-and-a-half-inch incision in his neck just beside his trachea; had dissected out the carotid artery, which was about the size of my index finger; and felt the plaque that had caused the decreased flow of blood to that side of his brain. From the outside of the artery, the blockage felt almost as hard as bone. I placed a clamp above and below the blockage and made a longitudinal incision to open the artery. The plaque was very firm, and it almost filled the cavity of the artery. I cleanly dissected it out from the lining of the vessel, flushed out the artery, and closed it with a fine suture. Such an operation is one of the most satisfying procedures a surgeon can perform.

That same afternoon I read an article in a medical journal about similar blockages. What it said made me commit to a change in my lifestyle—not eating my most favorite food.

I hadn't really thought about it before, but I considered it my job to clean out the arteries, not to teach patients how to prevent blockages in the first place. At least that was my mentality. I was saving patients from another stroke, and that was extremely satisfying, but the article pointed out that the biggest culprit behind such plaques is deposits of LDL cholesterol (the bad cholesterol we'll talk about later) within the wall of the artery. I knew that, but I hadn't dwelt on it. The article went on to say that saturated fat was the fat Americans ate the most that resulted in such blockages.

Then I read a statement that jumped out at me. Americans get the most saturated fat from cheese. It's not that cheese has more saturated fat than all other foods, but that we eat so much of it that the cumulative effect gives us more such fat than any other food. The cause of such blockages was something I had been doing to myself for years.

I could not believe what I was reading. I had just performed an operation I felt so good about, yet now I realized what I was doing to my own arteries. I reminded myself that cheese was my one favorite food. All my patients knew it was my favorite, and every Christmas gifts of cheese and cheeseballs completely filled my office desk.

I thought about that piece of plaque I had removed from the man's artery just hours ago, and I decided from a medical standpoint that I should never eat another bite of cheese in my life, that I had to kill the desire for it and break the habit. At that moment, I made that commitment, that promise to myself. That one medical article had awakened me to what was going on in my body and what I needed to do about it. I smiled as I closed the medical journal and placed it on my desk. I realized if I continued eating cheese after knowing what it could do to me, I would be foolish. I knew I was smarter than that, and that was the last of my cheese eating.

The next Christmas, I placed all my cheese presents on the office kitchen table and informed the staff they shouldn't eat them, but if any of them were foolish, they were welcome to do so. When I walked back into the kitchen an hour later, all the cheese was gone, but I didn't ask anyone to confess.

Your Revelation

Busy doctors may not have the time to go over everything patients need to change, so like my colleague, they simply prescribe medication; encourage patients to exercise, eat properly, and lose weight; and then send them on their way. But because you're reading this book, I feel sure you won't fall into the first category of patients that physician told me about—the patient who won't commit to making those lifestyle changes.

Reading one article made me commit to changing my lifestyle. My hope is that this book will inspire you to make that same commitment. Read and reread certain points that apply directly to you as you take on the challenge to do all you can to defeat diabetes. I believe you will look at your life a little differently once you know medically what is going on in your body as a diabetic, and what you can do to address the problem.

I can assure you, your doctor would love to have the time to teach you what medical research says about preventing or curing diabetes. Think of the time you spend reading this book as a conversation with your physician, explaining what's going on in your body and the specific changes you can make to improve your health.

Let this book help you make the lifestyle changes to prevent, delay, or improve diabetes, whichever stage you may be in. It will teach you changes you can make in your everyday life that will protect you from the health problems directly associated with diabetes. You will learn the significant effect diabetes has on your arteries, your heart, and your brain.

Two things are possible. One is that diabetes can be prevented, and two, that you can recover completely from type 2 diabetes.

It's More Than Sugar

Diabetes has impacts beyond simply not getting the glucose from the blood into the cells. The Centers for Disease Control points this out, showing many physical problems related to our arteries are associated with diabetes. Diabetes is listed as a separate risk factor for arterial disease. Additionally, one of the serious diseases that increase our chance of dying from a heart attack or stroke is *high blood pressure*. The CDC reports that 71 percent of diabetics have high blood pressure with a reading greater than 140/90. We'll talk later about how to read those numbers.

Another associated risk to your arteries feeding your heart is the role your *cholesterol* plays. The CDC report showed that 65 percent of diabetics have an increase in their "lethal," bad LDL cholesterol or were being treated for such. With bad LDL, you almost double your risk of heart attack and increase your risk for stroke one and a half times.

As we get to what you can do to prevent or reverse diabetes, don't forget all these additional problems associated with your arteries. You must address them as well.

Medical research points to two other major factors in defeating diabetes in addition to what you eat: *weight loss and exercise.* When you commit to weight loss and exercise, you increase the odds you will defeat diabetes. We'll review some of this research, so you can understand from a medical perspective why losing weight and exercising are essential for your success.

Learning about the relationship between diabetes and your heart and arteries will explain why the nurse I mentioned in the introduction to this book shed tears when her doctor told her being diagnosed as diabetic was the same as being told she had just had her first heart attack.

The Two Main Risk Factors in Developing Diabetes

Some of the best studies to evaluate how you can defeat diabetes are where the participants don't have diabetes—*yet*. These studies evaluate people who have what is called impaired glucose tolerance or are labeled prediabetic. They have higher-than-normal glucose but their numbers aren't high enough to be termed diabetic. Researchers follow them for several years to see who progresses to a diagnosis of diabetes. Some of the participants will make lifestyle changes and some won't. Then, after a period of time, the study will show whether lifestyle changes helped prevent diabetes. These studies provide excellent lessons for every diabetic.

One such study is reported in the *New England Journal of Medicine*. The research shows that *obesity and physical inactivity are the two main determinants of progression to the diagnosis of diabetes.* In this book you'll learn the specifics of how to combat these two risk factors, and it's interesting to know you can begin making changes right now to reduce those risks. In this study, the incidence of diabetes was reduced remarkably by losing weight and exercising. Even in people who didn't lose significant weight, exercise alone played a noteworthy role in the prevention of the impaired glucose progressing to full-blown diabetes.

Keep reading; you're going to learn how to fight both of those determinants.

The Relationship between Weight and Diabetes

Being overweight or obese may account for 80 to 85 percent of the risk of developing type 2 diabetes. Some studies suggest that obese people are up to eight times more likely to develop type 2 diabetes than those with a BMI of less than 22. One reason, it is thought, is because excess abdominal fat causes fat cells to release substances that cause inflammation around the cells that accept glucose. This relates to the insulin resistance. Researchers think this inflammation is a primary cause of the swelling within the keyhole that blocks the insulin key from fitting into the lock to unlock the cell door, which then allows the glucose to enter the cell normally.

Even diabetic organizations don't adopt just one diet, although most groups agree that following a weight-reducing diet plan will enhance weight loss. The most frequent recommendation most international organizations give for diabetic patients is to achieve and maintain a body mass index of less than 25, and we'll talk more about BMI indicators. But such a BMI places you in the normal range of body weight for your height.

The good news is that a 5 percent reduction in body weight followed by regular, moderate-intensity exercise could reduce your type 2 diabetes risk by more than 50 percent.

The bad news is pointed out in an article in the *Journal of the American Medical Association*. The report stated that *less than 20 percent of diabetics try to lose weight by eating fewer calories and exercising.* That is a sad, sad statement. If someone knows what the problem is and doesn't do anything about it, they are traveling down the wrong road. Weight loss is a "must" in defeating diabetes, but more is required. Other lifestyle changes go along with reaching your ideal weight. We will get into specifics later, but I want to preview some of the medical research to show you what you can do today to improve your condition.

You can read many opinions about what foods to eat. Some say to eat mainly fats and avoid carbohydrates, and some studies do show that avoiding carbohydrates will result in not having to take as much insulin.

Others say to make certain types of carbohydrates the majority of your diet. Again, we will get into specifics later, but note that there are good fats as well as bad fats and good carbohydrates as well as bad ones. Good carbohydrates are interwoven into fiber, which releases the glucose slowly, not triggering a massive release of insulin when they're eaten. Then the bad ones, called refined sugars, are in foods such as pastries, donuts, and cakes, and are absorbed quickly with a spike in sugar levels, which causes the insulin battle to take place.

Fats fall into similar categories. Bad saturated fats affect the arteries of your heart and brain, which can result in a heart attack, stroke, or high blood pressure. Good fats, called monounsaturated and polyunsaturated fats, are found in fish, nuts, and olive oil, and they protect the arteries.

The type and quality of fat and carbohydrates are more important than the total amount of each. To start you thinking about the foods you will eat, a report in the *Annual Review of Public Health* points out that eating polyunsaturated and monounsaturated fat rather than saturated and trans fats plays an important role in controlling your diabetes. The report emphasizes eating whole-grain foods, which contain fiber, rather than refined-grain foods. Last, it emphasizes a diet rich in fruits, vegetables, whole grains, poultry, and fish, but encourages you to avoid red and processed meats, as well as refined grains, as in white breads.

Once more, we will get into the specifics for a proper diet later, but this gives you a framework to begin thinking about your eating habits.

This study also makes a point about the beverages we drink. The authors referenced a study that showed that frequent consumption of sugar-sweetened soft drinks of one serving or more per day is associated with a 40 percent increase in diabetes risk. What to do is a no-brainer if you're diabetic. One twelve-ounce can of regular soda contains the equivalent of ten teaspoons of sugar. *Never consume any calories from beverages.*

This study affirms some lifestyle changes can place you into a low-risk group. These variables included a low BMI (body mass index of less than 25), a diet high in cereal fiber and polyunsaturated fat but low in trans fat and low glycemic load, as well as exercising moderately to vigorously for thirty minutes a day, most days of the week. It also shows that up to 91 percent of diabetes cases can be prevented with these lifestyle practices concerning weight, exercise, and diet.

Cement one of the study's conclusions into your mind: *obesity is the strongest risk factor for diabetes, and obesity control is clearly the key to diabetes prevention.*

The key to your success, then, is maintaining your weight loss for the rest of your life. The Cochrane Collaboration addresses this issue in detail. It first presents a positive side, and then the extremely negative results found by different studies on weight loss in people who were prediabetic as well as those with a diagnosis of diabetes.

Researchers reviewed nine studies with a total of 5,168 participants. The follow-up ranged from one to ten years. Weight loss was successful initially and showed significant decreases in diabetes and associated problems. The study showed that weight loss and control must be key goals for people with diabetes, and that weight loss improves insulin sensitivity and glucose control as well as cholesterol levels and blood pressure.

The researchers quoted the American Diabetes Association's recommendation that said, "Individuals at high risk for developing diabetes need to become aware of the benefits of modest weight loss and participating in regular physical activity." The report went on to show that once you commit to your diet and exercise program, you can expect an average loss of 8 percent of your initial body weight over three to twelve months.

This study emphasized weight loss as the most important factor for diabetics to control their disease, showing that such loss resulted in a turnaround from insulin resistance to insulin sensitivity, with a resultant improvement in glucose control. With better insulin sensitivity, there was also a decrease in LDL cholesterol, blood pressure, and overall early mortality.

Quality of life is our goal, and these reports show a significant improvement in quality of life by not having to deal with the problems associated with diabetes and being overweight.

Then the report gives what I think is its most significant sentence: "However, these benefits are thought to be clinically meaningful *only* if weight loss is sustained over time."

That is the point I want to emphasize. You will lose all the benefits you've gained if you don't maintain weight loss. The beauty of this book's plan is that it is easily sustainable for life. It's not a fad diet; it's a lifestyle you will live out of habit from now on. You will not regain weight because you'll have overcome your desire for the wrong foods and set up a personal exercise routine. Because of what you know, you will run from your old ways of living.

Now for the sad side of their report. After reviewing several studies where diabetics lost weight but regained it, the Cochrane Collaboration concluded that weight loss and metabolic control were achieved, but not maintained. That conclusion is confirmed by numerous other studies that show at least half of all weight loss is regained within a year.

That is a real slap in the face that ought to get your attention. Unless you develop proper lifestyle changes as you lose your excess weight, you won't maintain your weight loss.

To lose weight and maintain that loss, you must replace unhealthy habits with healthy ones. This means changing your future one step at a time, and in such a way that you can continue walking that same path for the rest of your life—*out of habit*, which is the main secret of this book. I'll introduce you to what not to eat, as well as the significance of your weight when winning the battle with diabetes. When you reach the end of this book, you will know how to practice habits that will make it easy to succeed as you eat properly, follow your exercise plan, and lose weight.

3. Medicine vs. Lifestyle Change

Diabetes can be treated in two ways: with medication and with lifestyle change.

As a physician, I can tell you it's terrible to have to treat patients without a medicine that can cure their illness. But no medication exists to cure diabetes. The only cure depends on the patient, not the doctor. That's a difficult reality for a physician to accept, knowing that diabetes is a major risk for heart attacks and strokes, which cause the clear majority of deaths in diabetic patients. Diabetes is also a leading cause of blindness, kidney failure, and amputations.

Your doctor most likely started you on medication once the diagnosis of diabetes was made. If you're overweight, or eat the wrong foods, or don't exercise, however, you can make changes that will allow that dose of medicine to be reduced or even eliminated.

Medication is often the primary treatment for diabetes. If you talk with diabetics on insulin, they will go into detail about how much they take every day. They know the exact date their doctor put them on insulin. They routinely check their glucose and take the proper dose to keep a certain amount of glucose in their bloodstream. They take and control the amount of all this medicine, and do nothing else, because of one of two things: (1) they don't know lifestyle changes can improve or reverse their condition, or (2) they *do* know lifestyle changes can make a difference, but they simply don't want to make them. Their doctor must keep adjusting medication to take care of what they won't take care of themselves.

Medication is not your best answer. And that leads us to the second treatment: lifestyle change. It's imperative that the importance of your diet, your weight, and your physical activity be understood, and then, that understanding is applied in the overall treatment of your diabetes. My goal in this book is not to just point out the problems of diabetes, but to propose solutions. I want to inspire you to develop lifestyle habits that transform how you live. Your actions will speak louder than your words.

Even prediabetics are usually placed on a medication to control the level of glucose in their blood. Your physician knows what is in store for you down the road unless something is done. The worsening of the glucose and insulin relationship is almost a certainty, because most diabetics don't understand what's going on in their bodies or realize that lifestyle changes could control the *progression* of insulin resistance.

That is why I want to show you what medical research tells us about diabetes. It is possible to prevent, stop, or reverse the diabetic process of the buildup of insulin resistance, which causes the pancreas to have to increase the amount of insulin it produces. Once you start on medication, you're trying to take control of your glucose/insulin relationship rather than relying on your body to control the process. You will never be able to regulate your glucose and insulin as well as your body can control it. No matter how many times you check your glucose and inject yourself with a proportional amount of insulin, you cannot control it nearly as well as your built-in body control system that properly works when you don't have diabetes. The goal is to increase the insulin sensitivity of your cells, which will allow more glucose into the cells, and thus require less insulin to be produced by the pancreas.

If you get no other insight from this book than understanding the importance of doing everything you can to maximize your own body's regulatory system, then it has achieved its mission.

What Research Tells Us

The *British Medical Journal* speaks to this importance in an interesting article. Researchers reviewed seventeen studies that involved over eight thousand participants who had impaired glucose tolerance. Their introduction states, "Individuals with diabetes have a life expectancy that can be shortened by as much as fifteen years, with up to seventy-five percent dying of macrovascular complications." The statement means that when your doctor says you have prediabetes or diabetes, your death could occur as much as fifteen years earlier than it might if you work to defeat your diabetes.

What would you pay to live a good, quality life fifteen years longer than you might because of your diabetes?

The study also points out that most diabetics will die because of coexisting risk factors that affect the arteries in their bodies and lead to heart attacks and strokes. If your doctor just told you that you have diabetes, or that you must increase your medication, or that your insulin resistance has progressed to the point that you now need insulin, those statements should motivate you to change. I hope they'll motivate you to read this book more closely.

Some of the studies reviewed in this report showed that *lifestyle changes are twice as effective as the most common medication used in treating diabetes.* Any way you look at it, these studies underscore the difference in making lifestyle changes versus taking medication. Medication that must be taken for life often has side effects. Even minor side effects, such as gastrointestinal problems, take on a greater importance when you realize you will deal with them for the rest of your life.

The conclusion of the report stressed the effectiveness of lifestyle versus medication in treating diabetes. Researchers pointed out that diabetes is fundamentally a lifestyle issue and asked a question you can answer for yourself: Should what is fundamentally a lifestyle issue be treated with a life-long course of medication?

That question is one of the most important I have read about when it comes to what to do if you've been diagnosed as diabetic. I'm not saying medication isn't needed or is not useful, but we should consider how much impact our lifestyles can have on diabetes outside of medication. Report after report shows that even patients on insulin get off their insulin completely with lifestyle changes, and many can drastically reduce it.

The problem becomes evident, however, when you ask diabetics which they think is the better treatment—medication or lifestyle change. Their answer is often given as if it's a no-brainer. "Medication, of course."

Metformin is a popular drug for the treatment of diabetes. It works by helping diabetics respond better to their own insulin, lowers the amount of sugar created by the liver, and decreases the amount of sugar absorbed by the intestines. But if you did a study on individuals who were prediabetic and placed a portion of them on medication and a portion of them on lifestyle changes, and then followed them several years to see which ones developed diabetes, the results would tell you a lot about how to prevent or treat diabetes.

Such a study was performed and then reported in the *New England Journal of Medicine*. It will open your eyes to what you can be doing as a prediabetic or a diabetic. Researchers worked with more than three thousand nondiabetic people who were overweight and had elevated blood sugar. They used a BMI of above 24 as their definition of overweight. Some participants were placed on a placebo tablet that had no medical function, some on metformin tablets, and the others on a lifestyle modification program with the goal of at least a 7 percent weight loss and at least 150 minutes of physical activity each week. The basic exercise was brisk walking thirty minutes a day, five days a week.

What researchers found was quite unbelievable from a medical standpoint. As mentioned earlier in this book, if you go to your doctor with elevated blood sugar, he or she will most likely place you on a medication as well as tell you about the need for diet, exercise, and weight loss. As we have also said, however, doctors don't have time to go into detail about how important these lifestyle changes are, especially compared to the medication they've just prescribed. That's why learning what medical research shows is so important. These specialized studies tell you in detail what the average doctor doesn't have the time to explain. The results of this particular study are a real wake-up call.

The average follow-up on this study's participants was 2.8 years. The group that made lifestyle changes reduced the incidence of diabetes by 58 percent, while the metformin medication group reduced the incidence of diabetes by just 31 percent. In other words, *lifestyle changes were twice as effective as the medication.* The report stressed that type 2 diabetes is preventable, and that prevention is preferable to developing diabetes and treating it with medication.

The conclusion of the study makes another important point about the effect of diabetes on the heart. These researchers stressed that "cardiovascular disease is the leading cause of death among patients with type 2 diabetes." Cardiovascular disease means disease of the arteries of the heart. Treatment with medication helps control the level of glucose in the blood, but it doesn't treat the associated problems that come with not exercising, eating foods that cause damage to arteries, and not losing excess weight.

If you're overweight, don't exercise, and eat foods that have a negative effect on your arteries, simply taking the medication that helps keep your glucose in line gives you a false sense of security. Unless you look at the entire picture of what diabetes is doing to your body, you're treating only a fraction of your problem. Doctors can give you medicine for your glucose, but they can't give you a pill that's a substitute for what you should eat and whether you exercise or lose weight. *You are the only one who can wholeheartedly treat your condition, not your doctor.*

The study concluded that type 2 diabetes can be prevented or delayed in persons with a high risk for the disease. It's extremely important that you develop a lifestyle program that will improve your life, for the rest of your life. You don't want to simply control your glucose with medication and risk living with all the associated complications and difficulties that go with diabetes. You want quality years to do what you want to do with your life. That takes a commitment to develop a healthy lifestyle.

Nothing good is going to come of your diabetes unless you commit to changing some of your lifestyle choices, unless you stop depending solely on medication. Always remember that the road you're on determines your destination. The diabetic road will eventually lead to a heart attack, stroke, damage to your kidneys or eyes, or to the possibility of the arterial disease in your lower extremities resulting in amputation. Don't just depend on medication to control your blood sugar. The dangers are much greater than blood sugar levels reveal.

I'm reminded of what my mother taught me and my brothers when we were in high school. So many times, when she was reminding us what time she and my father expected us home, she said, "Nothing good ever happens after midnight." I will never forget when one of my good friends had a few beers, wrecked his car, and ended up in the hospital for a week. I went to see him one afternoon. When I returned home and told my mother how terrible he looked and felt, lying in the hospital bed with casts on his arms, I was expecting an outpouring of sympathy from her.

Her response was a stern look and one question: "What time did he wreck his car?" All I could do was tell her the truth. "It was two o'clock in the morning." She didn't have to say another word, because she knew I understood.

I am not your mother, but I will tell you this: *nothing good happens from diabetes*. But you can make lifestyle changes to prevent it and, if you already have it, treat it—and they all need to be made before the midnight hour.

4. Understanding Insulin Resistance

Diabetes begins with having a little more sugar in your blood than normal. Early on, something begins to block the control panel that allows the insulin key to unlock the door that lets the glucose transfer from the blood into the cell. As time passes, there is more resistance at that cell door, resulting in not allowing the insulin to work properly.

The important factor to understand is that the real problem is the resistance to allowing the insulin to enter the cell. This is called, simply enough, insulin resistance. It takes more and more of the insulin keys to get the door unlocked. At first, everything seems okay. The pancreas produces more insulin to make up for the problem of that extra glucose. However, eventually the pancreas can't make enough extra insulin to take care of the excess glucose that can't get into the cells. That's when blood work shows your glucose is elevated and your doctor informs you that you have diabetes.

Insulin resistance has three causes that by now should be sounding familiar to you as we seek to understand diabetes. See if you fit into any one of the three categories. If so, then you need to pay extra attention to an article from *Public Health Nutrition*, which points out that the three causes of insulin resistance are inactivity, improper diet, and overweight.

Here's what the study found, in each category, about people who were insulin resistant but not yet labeled diabetic.

Exercise. Insulin resistance was lessened in those who undertook vigorous exercise and not in those who elected to be sedentary.

Diet. A high saturated fat intake was associated with higher insulin levels, higher glucose levels, higher insulin resistance, and higher risk of developing type 2 diabetes.

Diet. Poly and monounsaturated fat foods showed a lower risk of type 2 diabetes, lower glucose numbers, and lower insulin resistance.

Diet. A low intake of dietary fiber significantly increased the risk of type 2 diabetes. Researchers concluded that fiber reduces insulin resistance.

Weight loss. Weight is determined by what someone eats and whether they exercise. The authors of this report cite a study where the individuals who ate properly and exercised reduced their risk of diabetes by 58 percent over the people in the study who did not eat properly and exercise.

Studies like this put diabetes and insulin resistance into proper perspective. When I read them, I look closely at the summary of their significant findings. Here's the conclusion this study reached: *"Weight loss achieved by an increase in physical activity and dietary change including reduction in total and saturated fat and increased dietary fiber can reduce the incidence of diabetes."*

Understanding insulin resistance is the first step to understanding the primary problems that lead up to and cause full-blown diabetes. Diabetes is primarily a disease that centers on insulin resistance rather than insulin deficiency.

The problem isn't just too much glucose in the blood; it's the resistance of the cells of the body to letting insulin work as a key to open the cell door to let that glucose into the cell. We can measure the amount of glucose in our blood and see it is elevated, but the real culprit is that the insulin key doesn't work properly to unlock the cell door to allow the glucose to transfer from the bloodstream into the cell.

What Causes Insulin Resistance?

The question is this: What causes this resistance?

An article published in *Biochemical Journal* helps explain what exactly causes the lock on the cell door to swell, which then keeps the insulin key from functioning properly. Researchers studied individuals with different fat deposits and found an inflammatory response in the ones who had what is called visceral adipose tissue. This is the fat around your mid-abdomen, and it's prominent in people who have that fatty apron inside the front mid-part of their belly. Not to get too deep into the specifics, but what I think is good to learn from this study is that increased inflammation within anyone's body exists if extra fatty tissue is present.

This study reported that inflammation is the potential link between fatty tissue and insulin resistance. Researchers also showed that certain products produced by the fat tissue could cause an inflammatory response in the cells where insulin was trying to get glucose in. If you think of inflammation similar to taking sandpaper and rubbing it on the palm of your hand until it becomes reddened and begins to swell, you can imagine what a similar reaction could be on the walls of the cells insulin is trying to work in. Their study was complex in identifying the exact particles that adipose tissue produced that caused inflammation and increased resistance to insulin, but the study concluded that obesity-associated insulin resistance is related to inflammation as indicated by the accumulation of those specific particles.

An article published in the *New England Journal of Medicine* takes us a little deeper into how excess fat tissue is related to insulin resistance. I won't go too far into medical detail, but just enough for you to gain an understanding. Researchers showed that the normal glucose-insulin mechanism takes place mainly in muscle cells and liver cells. Normally, glucose goes from the blood into the cells and is stored there as glycogen, which can be broken back down into glucose as the body runs out of the normal amount of glucose in the blood. Whenever blood glucose becomes low and the body needs more for fuel, the stored glycogen breaks down into glucose and is used.

The study again pointed out that the beta cells in the pancreas produce the insulin that drives the glucose in the blood to enter the cells. But they also pointed out that, with diabetes, the early problem is that the cells become resistant to the insulin and more and more insulin must be produced. Researchers stressed that the primary reason the glucose level goes up is because of "insulin resistance" of that pathway into the cells. Only later does it become evident that the beta cells of the pancreas can't produce enough insulin to get the excess sugar into enough cells for the body to function. Their comment was that "insulin resistance predates beta-cell dysfunction."

Insulin resistance plays the key role in causing diabetes. Knowing that most of the action happens in muscle cells and liver cells makes it easier to understand how fatty tissue in these two locations can affect how insulin works and how extra fat can cause insulin resistance at these two locations. Basically, the study showed that as extra fat tissue accumulates in muscle and the liver, there is more resistance to insulin being able to work properly. It's as though the extra fat tissue within the cells acts like a "cut-off" switch that prevents insulin from unlocking the door properly.

Yes, the study showed that extra fat tissue is a cause of insulin resistance, but the most significant and exciting finding is what happens to insulin resistance if you lose weight. Their main conclusion showed that *insulin resistance is reversed after weight loss.*

Their study had one more significant finding, involving a subgroup of individuals who exercised. Researchers found them to have even better results in improving insulin resistance.

The final takeaway of the study is that *combining weight loss with exercise "is clearly the preferred medical therapy."*

Hopefully, the insights from these studies not only help you understand the danger of extra fatty tissue in your body but also encourage you to work to get every extra clump of adipose tissue out of your system, whether it's where you can see it in your mid-gut or hidden within your liver and muscles.

This study focused on the cause of insulin resistance, but its conclusion could have been summarized in four words of advice to diabetics: lose weight and exercise.

Insulin Resistance: A Review

Hopefully, you're beginning to understand the steps toward developing diabetes, and insulin resistance is the initial step. Most people with insulin resistance don't realize they have it. It is silent, causing no symptoms, and then one day they can be diagnosed as diabetic.

When I was in medical school, I realized I needed to go over my notes from each day's lecture at least three times to retain the knowledge. A quick review now is that, initially, something prevents the insulin from being able to transfer the glucose from your bloodstream into the cell. That leaves excess glucose in your blood, but the body sensors just tell your pancreas to put out more insulin, which it does. The extra sugar finally gets into the cells because of the extra insulin, but as the insulin resistance gets a little worse, your body must produce more insulin, and finally, even the extra insulin is unable to get the excess glucose moved into the cells.

At this point, your lab report shows your blood sugar is a little above normal but not high enough to be labeled diabetic. As time goes on, the pancreas produces all the insulin it can, but it isn't enough to keep the glucose level below the level when your doctor tells you you're diabetic.

An article in *Current Molecular Pharmacology* points out that insulin resistance is associated with overeating and inactivity. More importantly, the researchers quoted in the article tied being overweight with heart disease, saying, "Cardiovascular diseases are basically twins of obesity." That says it well. If you are overweight or obese, and are inactive as well, you're setting yourself up for heart failure—a heart attack, bypass surgery, or stents.

An article in the *New England Journal of Medicine* states it best: "Insulin resistance is present in most of the 69% of American adults who are overweight or obese." Extra fat plays a significant role in the mechanism that blocks the lock on the door of the cells. Having excess weight is an initial step in developing diabetes, and it also plays a role in a combination of other problems related to diabetes. These include the effect on our cholesterol, with low levels of the "hero" HDL cholesterol and an elevation of the "lethal" LDL cholesterol, as well as an increase in high blood pressure.

If we want those locks on the cell doors to be sensitive to the insulin key when it attempts to unlock the door to allow glucose into the cells, we need to banish excess weight.

Defeating Insulin Resistance

Now that we understand the role insulin resistance plays in the cause and progression of diabetes, it's even more important to learn how to combat this hidden factor most people don't realize about diabetes. Let's look at something you can do to wipe out the cause of the problem, because it's a consistent problem throughout all stages of diabetes.

Getting rid of excess adipose tissue is your initial step in fighting insulin resistance, but that's intertwined with another lifestyle change: combining exercise with weight loss. This is the very best strategy for decreasing insulin resistance.

Let's review another study that takes us one step further toward proving the significance of exercise in decreasing insulin resistance. This study was published in the journal *Diabetes Care*, and I know it will encourage you to exercise as you also change your eating habits to lose weight.

Researchers wanted to see if intense exercise improved insulin resistance more than lighter exercise. They studied two groups. One group worked on weight loss with diet alone, and the other group worked on weight loss with diet *plus* intense exercise. Researchers wanted to see if more aggressive lifestyle intervention is more beneficial. They based the intensity of the exercise on how rapid the participants' heartbeats were as they exercised twenty to thirty minutes a day at least five days a week. They set the intensity level above the 80 percent level of maximum heart rate. The formula used to figure the 80th percentile heart rate is to take the number 220 and subtract the person's age. That gives the maximum heart rate. Taking 80 percent of that result gives the goal they used in measuring the intensity of exercise.

Insulin sensitivity changed significantly in the intensive exercise group. If you count your pulse as you exercise, you may find that if you haven't exercised in the past, a brisk walk will get your pulse to the 80th percentile. As your heart muscle gets stronger, you will need to increase your walk to a slow trot to get there. The same principle applies to bike riding, swimming, elliptical training, or using a treadmill. I encourage you to consult with your doctor to see if you have any limitations for exercise, and then begin your personal workout.

Weight loss and exercise are the two essentials in combating insulin resistance and diabetes. Exercise is the number one tool in losing weight, but your diet is a coworker. The journal *Diabetologia* reported which factors could improve insulin sensitivity so the cells would accept glucose more easily. Their focus was on the foods eaten by diabetics, and their comment was that insulin sensitivity "improved with the diet rich in polyunsaturated fatty acids compared with the diet rich in saturated fatty acids." That simply means the saturated fat found in red meat, cheese, cream, butter, and fried foods should be avoided and the good polyunsaturated fat found in fish, nuts, olive oil, and avocado should be eaten instead.

A study reported in *Lancet* summed it up: unless you develop a healthy lifestyle, your insulin resistance—and diabetes—will worsen.

Running out of insulin is not the *cause* of diabetes; it's the *result* of diabetes.

5. Diabetes and Your Heart

Remember the nurse who teared up as she told me she'd just been diagnosed with diabetes, and that her doctor said being told she was diabetic was the same as being told she had just had her first heart attack? That story reveals the elephant in the room for most diabetics—although they aren't ignoring it as much as they aren't realizing it's even there. They don't know the strong correlation of diabetes to heart failure or a heart attack. This is the one significant finding in medical literature everyone who is prediabetic or diabetic needs to understand.

An article in the *Journal of the American Medical Association* reported a study that pointed out the close association of insulin resistance and the risk of heart failure. Researchers emphasized how diabetes and obesity are a double whammy against us. They estimated the morbidity caused by heart failure in a diabetic is four to eight times that of the general population.

Obesity is a prime risk factor for heart failure. *Diabetes* is also a risk factor for heart failure. *Insulin resistance* is a precursor of both diabetes and heart failure even before diabetes is evident.

One quote from this report is especially important to absorb: "Abdominal obesity is closely associated with insulin resistance." Losing the excess weight there is especially crucial to defeating diabetes.

The good news is that the same lifestyle changes you can make to defeat diabetes will also protect the arteries of your heart. I call that a win-win.

How Your Heart Figures In

When we moved into our new home years ago, a friend of mine gave me a housewarming gift. I didn't own a gun, not even a pistol, but he thought I should have some sort of protection since I was living out in the country. I opened the box and was surprised to find a small double-barreled shotgun neatly packed with wrapping paper. I took it outside and shot it a few times—until my shoulder hurt, and then I put it away, thinking I would never need it.

Then one night at about three o'clock our burglar alarm went off. My heart started racing. I jumped out of bed, found the shotgun, and my son and I began going from room to room. He opened closet doors as I wondered if someone was hiding behind each one. It wasn't too long before I heard the back doorbell ring. I went to the door and saw the county sheriff standing there. When he saw me and my shotgun, he started laughing—loudly.

"Doc." He pointed toward the gun. "Let me give you some

advice. If you ever catch someone in your house, march them out to your backyard, shoot them, and then drag them back into the house." He kept laughing as he looked at my firearm. "If you shoot that gun indoors, your ears will ring for two weeks."

I knew he was kidding about shooting someone, but I was glad to know how loud a shot inside would be.

I had known someone seemed to be in my house in the middle of the night, but I hadn't known two other things. One was that when the alarm went off, it also notified the sheriff's office. The other was that one of the sensors was connected to a door in the garage that had blown open.

I tell you that story to remind you that diabetes is not just a single-barrel problem; it's a triple one. Most everyone thinks of diabetes as simply a sugar issue. That's part of the problem, but not all of it. Defeating diabetes has a triple target: diabetes prevention, heart disease prevention, and Alzheimer's prevention. Diabetes must be shot at with three barrels of lifestyle changes—exercise, diet, and weight. If you don't do what will protect against the heart- and brain-related problems of diabetes, you're not fighting the whole fight.

Protecting the arteries in your heart and brain are of paramount importance in association with diabetes. If I could get only one idea across to diabetics, it would be that diabetes has a huge impact on the health of arteries. The three lifestyle barrels you need to work on in defeating diabetes are all associated with the health of your arteries.

In this chapter we'll focus on the arteries in your heart, and in the next chapter on the arteries in your brain.

An article in the *Annals of Internal Medicine* points out the importance of the arteries in your heart the best. Researchers followed participants who had abnormal glucose levels but did not yet have diabetes. They were divided into a group that lost 7 percent of their weight and exercised thirty minutes a day at least five days a week. The other group was given a common medication to control their glucose. After 3.2 years, they were evaluated to see which group had protected their heart better by having controlled their blood pressure, their cholesterol level, and insulin resistance.

The exercise weight-loss group had over twice the improvement the medicine-alone group did, with a reduction of 41 percent in the lifestyle change group versus a decrease of only 17 percent in the medication alone group.

The message of the study is that diabetics need to go beyond relying on medication to control diabetes. They also need to focus on preventing the associated heart risks that go along with diabetes. Defeating diabetes is more than glucose control. It means also addressing the problems that are so commonly associated with diabetes, and that involves weight, cholesterol, blood pressure, and activity.

An article from the *American Medical Association* compared two groups of people—one that ate a significant amount of fiber and one that ate very little fiber. The odds of developing insulin resistance were sevenfold greater in the group that ate the least amount of fiber.

One point in this study is extremely important: diabetes affects the small arteries as well as the large arteries of the body, and this arterial involvement accounts for most of the increased morbidity and mortality associated with type 2 diabetes.

If I could make that statement above flash in red, I would. Here's why: if a diabetic loses weight and exercises, their fasting plasma glucose will go down, their fasting serum insulin will improve, their "hero" HDL cholesterol will increase, their "lethal" LDL cholesterol will decrease, and both their systolic and diastolic blood pressure will improve. Weight loss and exercise address the glucose and improve heart health.

Diabetes = Heart Attack

An article published in *Acta Diabetologica* includes this eye-catching statement: "Diabetes is now considered a heart attack equivalent and, therefore, an aggressive, multifactorial, long-term intervention in patients with diabetes is critical." What the authors of this study are saying is exactly what this book is emphasizing, and what that diabetic nurse's doctor told her. You can't look at diabetes as only a sugar problem; you must look at where that diabetic path leads. The clear majority of diabetics die from heart disease.

Coronary heart disease (CHD) refers to disease of the arteries of your heart. As LDL cholesterol builds up in the walls of the arteries, bleeding and clots or plaque formation build up. This leads to a decreased flow of blood through that artery and subsequently less blood to the area that artery is supplying. The medical reports center on heart disease because that's the organ most commonly affected by a decrease in blood flow.

It's important, however, to understand that the problem occurring in the arteries in the heart also occurs in arteries throughout the body. When you read about heart attacks causing the most deaths of diabetics, a little further you will see an additional percentage of deaths and disabilities because of blockage of arteries in the brain, which results in strokes. (Again, we'll talk more about the arteries of the brain in the next chapter.) The same process occurs in the arteries of the legs. The number one cause of amputations of lower extremities is blockage of arteries in the legs of diabetics. So keep all the risk factors of diabetes in mind as you choose an eating plan.

This article makes some dietary suggestions for heart health:

- Lower consumption of red meat, processed meat, dairy products, egg yolks, butter, and margarine.
- For good fat in a diet, eat poultry, fish, nuts, and olive oil.
- For protein in a diet, mainly eat fish, peas, beans, nuts, or poultry.
- Avoid carbohydrates in refined grain and emphasize carbohydrates such as fruits, vegetables, peas, beans, and whole grains such as cereal.

There are good carbohydrates linked to fiber and bad refined carbohydrates that allow more glucose into your blood. And remember, there are good fats and bad fats. Stop eating bad fats and replace them with good ones. Your choice makes all the difference, as the article cited above puts it clearly: "Replacement of saturated fat with monounsaturated fat is associated with a 3-fold greater reduction in coronary heart disease than that obtained by replacement of saturated fats with carbohydrates." The good fats are found in fish, olive oil, and nuts. The bad fats are in red meat, cheese, egg yolks, cream, butter, and most fried foods.

Cholesterol Matters

When you finish reading this book and get started, you will have developed an eating plan that will not only control the glucose in your system but also protect your arteries. I want you to understand the connection of having diabetes and ending up with a heart attack or stroke. To do so, you need to not only know how carbohydrates affect your body but also the importance of your cholesterol numbers.

Let's look briefly at the most common cholesterol particles reported on your blood work—the LDL cholesterol and the HDL cholesterol particles—and how they impact your arteries.

Getting a splinter in your finger is the best illustration of what happens when LDL cholesterol gets into the walls of your arteries. I call the reactive process that takes place the "splinter syndrome." The spot where the splinter is embedded begins to swell and turn red. The surrounding tissue considers that splinter a "foreign body," and if the splinter doesn't come out, your body's natural response is to develop a wall of scarring tissue around it. The initial swelling around the splinter is the result of the body pouring fluid into the area. The fluid is filled with soldier-type cells, called macrophages, that attack the splinter. Many times there is even bleeding into this swollen battlefield, and the finger turns red and more swollen.

Finally, one of two things happens. The resulting inflammation can be so fierce that it swells and the fluid breaks through the skin and drains out. An example of this is a boil that ruptures and drains from the battleground tissue to the outside. Or after the battle against the foreign body splinter reaches its height, healing begins to take place. The body sends cells called fibroblasts that begin to lay down fibers that join to form a healing scar throughout the battlefield.

This scar tissue is not the normal kind of tissue once there. Scar tissue is firmer and harder and isn't pliable. You can palpate the thickened, hardened area of scar tissue forming just under the skin's surface, and that scar remains—fixed, thickened, firm, hard, and swollen. If another splinter enters the skin in that same area, another battle takes place, and the resulting scar area gets larger and larger. After repeated battles, calcium can become a part of the healing, and the plaque buildup is even firmer and harder.

A similar process happens in the walls of your arteries. I like to think of sugar as the beginning cause of inflammation. Once again using sandpaper as an illustration, I visualize sugar as a piece of sandpaper that rubs the walls of arteries raw, which allows for easier access into the wall of the arteries of the LDL cholesterol splinters. The initial step is that of inflammation. LDL cholesterol is the splinter that gets through the lining of the artery and into the media, the middle portion of the arterial wall. However, there's a difference between getting a splinter stuck in your finger and getting an LDL cholesterol splinter stuck in the wall of your artery.

If you stick your hand into the middle of a thornbush and get stuck, you won't stick your hand in again because you felt the pain of the prick. The problem with the LDL cholesterol splinter syndrome is that you don't feel the splinters going into your arteries. These splinters get through the lining wall of your arteries and cause the battle to begin, and the wall of your artery reacts much like your finger does to a splinter. The area can become so inflamed that there is bleeding with the inflammatory reaction, and it can rupture through the lining into the lumen of the artery. A clot forms and plugs the entire artery at that point.

Or the arterial wall can stay intact and the splinter battleground ends in a healing process. But the scars of battle remain. The enlarged scar formation protrudes into the lumen of the artery, and the result is a partial blockage of the flow of blood through that area (like crimping a straw). This is what is commonly referred to as plaque buildup. The next time an LDL cholesterol splinter gets stuck in the same area, the process repeats itself. The secondary battleground either pops open and causes a clot to form inside the artery, or it heals again and bulges even more into the inside of the artery. The result is more plaque buildup. This secondary plaque protrudes even farther into the lumen of the artery, causing the flow of blood to be even less to the heart muscle downstream.

It's imperative to keep your LDL cholesterol low. But how you get there is more important than just getting the numbers down. You can be fooled if you're only looking at the numbers. Taking medication alone, without lifestyle changes, isn't a guarantee that you're doing all you can to protect your arteries. You should work on your LDL score as you would a golf score—the lower the better. Think of saturated fat in food being the main cause of your LDL cholesterol becoming elevated. Think of it every time you want to eat red meat, cheese, egg yolk, cream, butter, or any fried foods.

The other side of the coin from the lethal LDL cholesterol is HDL cholesterol. HDL stands for high-density lipoprotein cholesterol. Think of the *H* as standing for "hero" or "healthy." This is the good cholesterol number you'll be attempting to get as high as possible. HDL cholesterol protects you by battling the LDL cholesterol. Here's an easy way to visualize how this works:

Think of an HDL cholesterol particle as a patrol car that floats through the bloodstream, looking for LDL cholesterol criminals. Imagine the HDL cholesterol patrol car pulling up to an area where LDL cholesterol "splinters" are getting into the wall of an artery. The HDL cholesterol patrol car picks up several splinters, carries them to the liver, and then deposits them there to be disposed of. The liver takes the LDL cholesterol particles and passes them out of the body in the bile. While the liver is working to place this excess LDL cholesterol into the process of forming bile, the HDL cholesterol "patrol car" particle is on its way back to the arteries, where it picks up some more LDL cholesterol to transport back to the liver.

You want as few LDL splinters as possible and as many HDL patrol cars as possible.

How do you do this? Think of the saturated-fat foods as raising your LDL cholesterol. Think of exercise and losing weight as raising your HDL cholesterol. Eat right. Exercise. Get to your ideal weight.

As you can now begin to understand, diabetes is a much larger concern than just trying to control your blood sugar. The foods you eat, the exercise you do, and the weight you carry all affect your cholesterol, which harms your arteries if it's too out of balance.

The same lifestyle risk factors that contribute to diabetes also put your arteries at risk, which affects your heart and brain. All these systems are intertwined. When you make changes to defeat diabetes, those changes will protect your heart and brain health as well.

Now let's turn to your brain.

6. Diabetes and Your Brain

This will probably be shocking to most diabetics because it hasn't received the emphasis it should have, but diabetes plays a big part in leading you toward the most dreaded disease in America—Alzheimer's.

Plaque buildup within the artery wall constricts the blood flow and eventually can block the artery. In a nutshell, this explains the relationship between diabetes and Alzheimer's. The blockage affects the blood flow to each cell of your brain. The inflammation and blockage of your arteries may reside in your larger vessels, as in your carotid arteries, which you can feel on each side of your windpipe. But similar blockages can also occur in the smaller arteries that directly feed the oxygen and nutrients to those neurons within your brain.

The brain is only 2 percent of our body's total weight. But it uses 20 percent of the oxygen we breathe and 20 percent of the nutrients we take in from food. Your heart and arteries are crucial in getting the needed oxygen and nutrients to each neuron of the brain. So stroke is not the only problem diabetes sets you up for within the brain.

The following two statements should be red alerts to anyone who is diabetic or who has a friend or family member who is.

- *Diabetes doubles your chances of developing Alzheimer's dementia.*
- *Diabetes accelerates progression from its early stage, called mild cognitive impairment, to full stage-3 Alzheimer's dementia by three years.*

Diabetes affects your arteries, which causes a decrease of blood flow to your brain. The excess insulin produced because of being diabetic can lead to an inflammatory response in the cells in the brain, and inflammation is one of the contributing causes of Alzheimer's. Being diabetic is a double hit for Alzheimer's. One, it has a negative effect on your arteries, being one of the vascular risk factors that cause a decreased blood flow to the nerve components of your brain. Two, it's a significant cause of the inflammatory response within the cells within the brain.

As we've said, you can do much more to beat diabetes besides taking medication. And as we discuss Alzheimer's, remember that each of the lifestyle changes you can make related to diabetes is also directly related to what is going on in the brain. This can be a most powerful incentive to help you commit to changing your lifestyle. Making wise choices concerning your diet, exercise, and weight will not only affect your diabetes but also decrease your risk of Alzheimer's.

Many medical journal articles highlight the correlation between the health of your arteries and the health of your heart and brain. They commonly conclude that *what is good for the heart is good for the brain*. What makes this so relevant is that, medically speaking, diabetes is listed as one of the risk factors for disease of your arteries. This is one link diabetes has with Alzheimer's. The *Diabetes Heart Study* pointed out that because the brain uses such a high proportion of total blood in your body, it's obvious that anything that affects the arteries that carry so much blood to your brain will also affect how your brain functions.

You don't want anything blocking the flow of blood to the nerve cells of your brain. This study investigated the correlation between the health of the heart and the scores on mental testing used to evaluate the person's cognition in relation to symptoms that could lead to Alzheimer's. Here is what the researchers found.

Even before symptoms became apparent, the investigators measured the amount of plaque within the walls of the arteries in the heart. Then seven years later, mental testing was performed using the cognitive tests for following Alzheimer's, which measured memory, executive function, and how fast test subjects processed different situations. The study found that the individuals with the greater amount of plaque in their arteries when the study began scored lower on the mental testing than did the people with the least amount of blockage of the arteries in their heart. This is a great reminder that what is good for the arteries of the heart is good for the arteries of the brain. Diabetes plays a significant role in the health of your arteries within your brain.

The relationship of diabetes to Alzheimer's is a relatively recent finding, and, as I said, hasn't been as emphasized to the general public as it should be. An article from the Alzheimer's Association discusses the importance of doing all you can to protect your arteries if you have diabetes. The article states that controlling the risk factors that affect the health of your arteries can reduce your chances of Alzheimer's dramatically.

Diabetes Is Not a Stand-Alone Disease

The article also points out that most of these arterial risk factors of high LDL cholesterol, being overweight, not exercising, diabetes, and high blood pressure are interrelated and connected to a general, overall unhealthy lifestyle. Minimizing these risk factors even reduces the chance of developing certain common cancers.

We need to address these intertwined lifestyles simultaneously. I especially like the conclusion, which the authors of this report put in bold print, highlighting diabetes as one of the causative factors: "The public should know what the science concludes: certain healthy behaviors known to be effective for diabetes, cardiovascular disease, and cancer are also good for the brain health and for reducing the risk of cognitive decline."

Understanding Blood Flow to the Brain

What causes a decreased blood flow to the brain? The arterial problem so closely associated with diabetes is caused by inflammation and blockage of your arteries. The blockage part is primarily caused by the associated health problems of diabetes, which affect your arteries, allowing plaque buildup. Being overweight increases your LDL cholesterol as well as decreases your HDL cholesterol. Being sedentary does the same. And eating the wrong foods causes a rise in your LDL cholesterol.

The initial step is inflammation, resulting in the wall of the artery becoming swollen with excess fluid, and with special cells sent into the battlefield to fight the LDL. The result is often plaque buildup within the wall, which constricts the blood flow and eventually can block the artery. The blockage affects the blood flow to each cell of your brain. The inflammation and blockage of your arteries may reside in your larger vessels, such as your carotid arteries in your neck.

Even more important is that similar blockage can occur in smaller arteries that directly feed the oxygen and nutrients to those neurons within your brain.

It is an accepted figure that over 80 percent of diabetics will die from heart disease because of disease of the arteries. It is also accepted that diabetes and heart disease are definitely associated.

Studying what goes on in the heart just before heart attacks also shines some light on the relationship of diabetes and Alzheimer's. Angina is a term used to describe chest pain caused by the heart muscles not getting enough blood supply. It is a loud warning that a heart attack is imminent because the arteries are not getting enough oxygenated blood to the heart muscles.

An article in the *Journal of the American Medical Association* noted that angina is associated with a more rapid mental decline once Alzheimer's is diagnosed. This study listed diabetes as one of the arterial risk factors that causes the chest pain of angina to develop. Also listed in addition to diabetes were other factors we've been discussing as related to diabetes, including high LDL cholesterol, high blood pressure, and the presence of atherosclerosis, which is the buildup of plaque in the larger arteries of the body, such as the carotid arteries, which supply the brain. All these factors that cause the heart pain associated with angina have been associated with an increased risk of Alzheimer's and are also risk factors associated with diabetes.

The takeaway of this study is that the more disease an Alzheimer's patient has in the arteries, the faster and worse Alzheimer's symptoms become.

Now, knowing the relationship diabetes has with Alzheimer's and the associated disease of your arteries, you also know the importance of protecting your arteries through the three lifestyle choices that can defeat diabetes: diet, exercise, and weight control. This study also showed that even if you do experience symptoms of Alzheimer's, it's never too late to change your lifestyle to guard against these arterial risk factors and slow the process of more beta-amyloid plaques forming within your brain. I like the conclusion of this study: "Treatment of vascular risk factors is associated with slower decline in Alzheimer's disease."

The same is true with diabetes: lifestyle changes in diet, weight control, and exercise are effective in defeating diabetes as well as slowing your odds of developing Alzheimer's. Changing your habits can address all these arterial risk factors.

Don't Double Your Odds for Alzheimer's

This eye-opening statement appears in a report in the *American Journal of Geriatric Pharmacotherapy*: "If you have diabetes you have doubled your chance of developing Alzheimer's." That is an alarming statistic about the association of diabetes and Alzheimer's. The connection is tied to the effect diabetes has on your arteries and heart, and in turn, the effect your heart has on your brain. The report gives a synopsis of the overall health of your arteries and why it's so important to defeat diabetes as well as fight high blood pressure, overweight, and inactivity. All these factors are directly related to diabetes, and if you protect your arteries by defeating diabetes, you will also be protecting your brain from developing Alzheimer's. Here are some motivating statistics from this report:

- If you've had a stroke, you are three and a half to six times more likely to develop Alzheimer's.
- If you have high blood pressure in midlife, you have four times the risk of developing Alzheimer's.
- If you have diabetes, you have doubled your chance of developing Alzheimer's.
- If you are obese in midlife, you have an increased risk of Alzheimer's in later life.
- If you regularly exercise, you can reduce your risk of developing Alzheimer's.
- If you regularly exercise even after symptoms of Alzheimer's have begun, even if you are over sixty-five years of age, you may prevent the progression of mental decline normally seen with Alzheimer's.

Diabetes and the Five Risk Factors of Alzheimer's

The medical journal *Neurology* made a sad statement concerning the arterial risk factors that increase your chances of Alzheimer's. These include diabetes, elevated LDL cholesterol, excess weight, being sedentary by not exercising, and high blood pressure. What researchers found was this: the combination of all these risk factors could increase the likelihood of dementia more than sixteenfold. These are the same risk factors associated with diabetes alone.

With such a statement as this, a loud alarm should be going off in your mind—*right now.* Can you hear it?

The five known primary risk factors for Alzheimer's all affect the arteries that supply the blood to the brain. Diabetes is one risk factor, and it is known to be intermingled with the rest. These "nasty five" are factors you can control with lifestyle choices. Each affects the health of your arteries, which in turn determines whether your brain is receiving the essentials to carry on normal mental function. If you are diabetic, in addition to diabetes, do you have any of the other risk factors in this list?

1. Diabetes
2. Elevated LDL cholesterol
3. Physically inactive
4. Overweight or obese
5. High blood pressure

Each of these factors enhances your chance of developing Alzheimer's, but each is intertwined with the others.

Now, let's look ahead at the lifestyle choices that lessen your risk of Alzheimer's. They are the same ones that defeat diabetes, and they should be familiar to you by now.

1. Exercise
2. Proper diet
3. Ideal weight

Lifestyle Correlations of Diabetes and Alzheimer's

Exercise

In reviewing the medical literature concerning diabetes, I concluded that exercise plays an extremely important role in defeating diabetes. It is so important that I rank exercise as the number-one lifestyle change for you to begin working on. Exercise has also been shown to be significant in relation to Alzheimer's. Being diabetic is a negative factor for developing Alzheimer's disease, and being sedentary—not exercising—is a large part of that. An article in *Lancet Neurology* reported on a collection of studies concerning diabetes, exercise, and Alzheimer's, and the significance of exercise or the lack of it.

The authors of the study concluded that being physically inactive contributed to the largest proportion of Alzheimer's disease in the United States. They based their conclusion on evidence that exercise played an important role in how closely associated it is with other risk factors for dementia. They also pointed out that individuals who don't exercise are more likely to have diabetes and high blood pressure and be obese—all of which mark a greater risk of dementia.

As you can see, once again, we're not dealing with a single contributory factor for diabetes or Alzheimer's; the risk factors are intertwined. If you begin a personal exercise program, you will be astonished at how many different aspects of your health improve. Exercise is a prime component in losing weight, as well as preventing or improving diabetes and high blood pressure.

Their report concluded that exercise and the associated risk factors were "all inter-related and probably contribute to Alzheimer's disease largely through a vascular mechanism." That reiterates that the health of your arteries causes better blood flow to the neurons of your brain. I keep reminding you, the health of your arteries plays a significant role in diabetes.

Another article in the *Journal of the American Medical Association* compared individuals who were physically inactive to those who exercised. The study went on for fifteen years, and researchers concluded that being inactive gave people a 50 percent greater chance of developing Alzheimer's.

A similar article in the journal *Neurology* compared people who were the least active versus the ones who exercised at least two times a week. Now, twice a week is not a lot of exercise, but the results were still astonishing. The ones who were sedentary were 60 percent more likely to develop Alzheimer's than the ones who exercised. Another study on exercise published in the journal *Neurology* used a device worn on the arm of the participants that gave a continuous measurement of their exercise activity. Those with lower overall physical activity had two negative results. One was a higher risk of Alzheimer's and the second was a faster rate of "cognitive decline." The study concluded that "low physical activity is deleterious to the brain." (I looked up the word *deleterious* and here are some definitions I found: harmful, poisonous, deadly, lethal, damaging, destructive, and injurious.) Results like this should motivate you to get moving. You can even watch sports or a favorite show on television while you're on a treadmill or elliptical machine.

Time and again, research shows the importance of exercise in lowering your chance of developing Alzheimer's as well as improving diabetes. Don't forget: from a medical standpoint, it's extremely important to have a personal exercise routine to fight against both diabetes and Alzheimer's.

Weight

Being overweight or obese is one of the main factors for an increased risk of developing Alzheimer's as well as diabetes. There's also a close relationship between diabetes, being overweight, having high blood pressure, and an elevated LDL cholesterol. The triad of being overweight, having high blood pressure, and having diabetes all affect the health of your brain as related to Alzheimer's.

An article in *Archives Neurology* reported on a study in Finland that looked at three important risk factors (high LDL cholesterol, high blood pressure, and obesity) and determined how much risk each was in the development of Alzheimer's. The findings showed that the people who had all three of these risk factors increased their chances of developing Alzheimer's six times greater than someone without these factors. When they broke them down to individual risks, they found an additive effect, with each of them increasing the risk of Alzheimer's by approximately two times.

High Blood Pressure

As mentioned before, over 80 percent of diabetics are over-weight. People who have both these health risks—diabetes and excess weight—also often have high blood pressure. We talk about these three factors of diabetes, overweight, and high blood pressure together because they are so interrelated. Maybe you're diabetic but haven't been diagnosed with high blood pressure, but let me just say, it could be on its way without your even being aware of it.

Here's a quick review of what your blood pressure numbers mean:

The first number in a blood pressure reading is called the systolic number. Imagine your heart squeezing down and pumping a large amount of blood into your arteries. They begin to bulge and expand under the pressure. The amount of pressure pushing on the walls of the arteries is called the systolic pressure.

When the heart muscle finishes its contraction, it goes into a resting stage as the heart is being refilled with blood. When this happens, the amount of blood flowing through your arteries is reduced, which then reduces the pressure against the arterial walls as they relax. That relaxed pressure is called the diastolic blood pressure number.

Normally, those two numbers would read 120 over 80 (120/80). You would not be classified as having hypertension, high blood pressure, until your pressure reads 140/90 or above. But the problem lies in between having a "normal" pressure and having "high blood pressure." Many people's pressure is neither normal, nor labeled as high blood pressure. They are borderline. Their blood pressure measures somewhere above the 120 systolic mark, yet below the 140 line. The same with the diastolic number. It's above the norm of 80, but below the 90 measurement. This is called prehypertension.

Being in this category should alarm you. And recently, the diagnosis of high blood pressure has been changed to anything over 120/80. All that says is that high blood pressure is a progressive condition, and we should be doing all we can to keep it in the completely normal range.

You may be diabetic and overweight and not have high blood pressure, but if you are obese you are probably on the route toward hypertension.

Your weight is an indicator of so much more than heaviness. Most obese people are sedentary. They become couch potatoes. I remind you, you may not be labeled obese, but if you're overweight, you may as well look at yourself as being "preobese" and start following the guidelines we set for weight loss. If you work on losing weight, you'll be working on the prevention of Alzheimer's as well as defeating diabetes.

The takeaway from the current research on Alzheimer's is this: it's important to develop the lifestyle choices you're learning from this book to protect the arteries in your brain as well as in your heart. Defeating diabetes is a great form of Alzheimer's prevention, and prevention supersedes any treatment known for Alzheimer's.

7. The Midlife Years

Are you in your midlife years of forty to sixty?

As with most things relating to your health, the earlier you begin prevention, the better. Multiple studies have examined risk factors in midlife of certain patients and followed them into later life. Researchers were able to identify which factors predicted which people were more prone to develop Alzheimer's than others. In other words, someone who had artery-damaging risk factors in midlife was much more prone to develop Alzheimer's later than the individuals who did not have those problems.

People who were diabetic in midlife were more prone to also have a higher LDL cholesterol or high blood pressure, or to be overweight and not exercise. When followed into later life, they were found to have a higher incidence of Alzheimer's than those who did exercise, who ate properly to keep their LDL cholesterol low, who were at an ideal weight, and who did not have diabetes or high blood pressure. Diabetes is the foundational base of so many problems associated with the health of your arteries and your brain, which lead to Alzheimer's.

Reports in some of the leading medical journals offer these insights into how your lifestyle choices, especially in *midlife*, affect whether you develop Alzheimer's in later life. A variety of specific studies published in the journals *Lancet Neurology*, the *Annals of Internal Medicine*, *Neurology*, and the *Archives Neurology* all point out that your chances for having Alzheimer's in later life are greater if in midlife certain health measurements directly related to diabetes are abnormal. These include your blood pressure being elevated or your BMI (body mass index) being elevated. Being overweight or obese is not good. Your chances are worse if your LDL cholesterol is elevated during your midlife years. The sentence that jumped out at me in the journal *Neurology* pinpointed the connection diabetes has with Alzheimer's: "Diabetes is associated with an increased risk of Alzheimer's throughout life but is even stronger when it occurs in mid-life." That's why you want to begin the battle against diabetes as young as you can.

Another study published in the journal *Neurology* emphasizes the importance of beginning the defeat of diabetes and Alzheimer's as early as possible, even during the early years of midlife. It described how artery risk factors in midlife relate to the risk of Alzheimer's in late life. Diabetes is one of the significant risk factors the authors of this study are referring to.

The investigation studied over eight thousand participants between the ages of forty and forty-four. Their medical records were examined to determine who developed dementia. Then these participants' midlife medical records were reexamined and correlated to see if those who had artery-disease risk factors in their midlife period developed dementia in later life.

What researchers found was astonishing. They discovered that "the presence of multiple cardiovascular (arteries of the heart) risk factors at midlife substantially increases risk of late-life dementia in a dose dependent manner." Significantly, they listed specific artery risk factors with diabetes—heading the list: diabetes, high cholesterol, high blood pressure, and smoking—and stated that they were each associated with an increased risk of dementia in later life. The study reported the statistics by each risk factor:

- Diabetes—46 percent more likely to have dementia
- High cholesterol—42 percent more likely
- Obesity in midlife—3.1 times more likely
- Overweight—2 times more likely
- High blood pressure—24 percent more likely
- Smoking—26 percent more likely

If you have diabetes, you are much more prone to have high LDL cholesterol, be overweight or obese, and have high blood pressure. So as we study the numbers reported in this study, correlate any additional medical issues you have with what they found.

Here are the statistics about dementia risk factors:

- One of the above—27 percent more likely to develop dementia
- Two of the above—70 percent more likely

- Three of the above—200 percent or two times more likely
- Four of the above—237 percent more likely

Note that being obese is the worst of all. So many other risk factors for your arteries are linked to being overweight. Remember that the number one association with individuals who are diabetic is *being overweight*.

Every item in the list is a risk factor for disease of your arteries. This sounds a loud alarm on the significance the health of your arteries plays in Alzheimer's as well as diabetes. Diabetes has a direct correlation with each of these risk factors mentioned, except for smoking. The good news is you can control these risk factors to not only defeat diabetes but to fight against Alzheimer's.

And the earlier you start, the better.

What Is the Exact Cause of Alzheimer's?

I wish we did, but no one knows the exact cause of Alzheimer's. We know that the more beta-amyloid protein that builds up around the neurons in the brain, and the more tangled tau protein that is within those cells, the greater the symptoms. All the above risk factors are associated with an increased buildup of beta-amyloid. But what exactly causes the excess beta-amyloid? Is it the actual beta-amyloid that *causes* the problem? Or is it something else that simply *results* in too much beta-amyloid to be in those locations? Normally, a certain amount of beta-amyloid is produced within the brain and a certain amount of it is removed into the bloodstream. So is too much beta-amyloid produced?

Or is there a blockage of the drainage process resulting in too much left in the brain?

An interesting article published in *Experimental Gerontology* reports on a study done in Austria, which shines some light on this question. This study points out some possibilities. One, the artery disease risk factors of having diabetes, high cholesterol, and disease of the small arteries around the neurons may cause damage to the cerebrovascular system—the cluster of the small arteries feeding the neurons—that could cause small strokes in the area. Or those same risk factors could cause a hindrance of the beta-amyloid clearance where it does not cross the blood-brain barrier where it gets back into the blood to be carried away. Such a disruption would result in an increase of beta-amyloid left in the brain tissue.

Whatever the cause, paying attention to the health of your arteries will make a difference for your brain.

PART 2

DEFEATING DIABETES:

LIFESTYLE CHOICES FOR YOUR HEALTH

8. Habits

"Type 2 diabetes is preventable." That's what an article published in *Diabetes Care* journal states. *How?* you may ask. The study's answer was this: by lifestyle intervention. This article gives numbers on prevention of diabetes, but the same concept applies to those who already have the disease. Let's see what will help not only in the prevention of diabetes but also the prevention of progression and help in reversing the problem.

The lifestyle interventions they studied involved four items: reduce body weight, reduce dietary and saturated fat, increase dietary fiber, and increase physical activity. They divided the individuals in their study into two groups, one that worked on the interventions and one that did not. The overall outcome was that the intervention group reduced their risk of diabetes by 58 percent as compared to the group that did not make the lifestyle changes.

A negative side to their study must be considered. This study measured the participants' weight at one year and three years. They lost an average of ten pounds at the end of the first year but had regained 25 percent of it at the end of three years. The same sad aspect of numerous other studies on weight loss is that many participants regain some or much of their weight.

If you apply what you learn in this book, you will not regain weight. If you develop a proper eating lifestyle as you lose weight, you will be able to maintain that ideal weight for the rest of your life because you will have changed your eating habits. The less regained, the better the effectiveness at defeating diabetes. Our goal is going to be 0 percent regain. Never forget this study's conclusion: *Type 2 diabetes is preventable. It is preventable by lifestyle changes.*

"If Only I Had Known"

So many patients say if only they had known their condition would end up the way it did, they would have changed their lifestyle habits years ago.

I will never forget this event when I was a surgical resident in training. An overweight diabetic patient was in the emergency room, lying on a stretcher with his left leg and foot exposed. I looked at the worst ulcer on an ankle and foot I had ever seen. Both of his legs were swollen, but the left was reddened up to his knee. The ulcer was so inflamed I had to wonder how long he had waited before deciding to come to the hospital. The yellow purulent material was slowly draining from the silver-dollar-sized ulcer.

The senior resident told me, "It's going to take an above-knee amputation. If you take it off below his knee, the wound will never heal, and two months later you'll be taking him back to the OR for a secondary above-knee amp."

I remember hoping we could do a below-knee procedure, so the prosthesis would be much simpler, but the senior resident made sense. Even if we left the wound open, it would never heal. He was diabetic.

I kept wondering why that patient hadn't decided to do something about his health before the arteries were so blocked with plaque that there wasn't enough blood flow to keep his left leg alive. What makes one person decide to make changes to prevent having their leg amputated, yet another ends up in the emergency room wishing they had?

That emergency room event was years ago. I'm not sure the patient had known he could make lifestyle changes that would prevent his leg amputation. If he had known about all the medical research you're reading, though, would he have changed the way he was living?

Unfortunately, it was too late for him to save his leg. Nothing he or we could do would save his arteries and allow his foot to survive. Don't wait until that day when nothing whatsoever can be done to prevent such a catastrophe.

It's All about Habits

We do so many things throughout the day because of habits. We've made a habit of what foods we eat. Our weight rises instead of falling because we haven't developed the habit of exercising.

One of the main reasons people change habits is because some physical event gets their attention. Something must be done, and only they can make it happen.

One morning I looked at my phone and realized someone had called at 5:42 a.m. As I listened to the voice mail,

I realized it was from a gentleman I had known for several years but had not kept up with recently. He was letting me know he was on his way to the operating room to have surgery on an artery in his heart. "I'm going to change a lot of what I do from now on. I'm not going to let this happen again" was his extremely serious statement to me as we talked later that day.

I remembered him being diabetic and overweight, and I knew he had tried to get his diabetes under control. He had lost some weight, changing his eating some, but mainly by what he called "moderation" of the bad foods. He regained the weight. It kept going through my mind that his situation was the main reason people change their lifestyles—they receive a wake-up call from their bodies and decide to listen to it.

I have a friend I see each winter because we have condo units next door to each other. Last year, he asked if I had a copy of my book *Prescription for Life* that he could read. He had experienced a health issue and had made the decision to change his lifestyle choices for eating, exercising, and weight control. He wanted to know the most effective way of doing it, one that medical research confirms. Of course, I gave him a copy of my book to begin his journey.

I couldn't believe my eyes a year later. I hardly recognized him. All his excess fat had disappeared, his face and neck were almost skinny, and he looked ten to twelve years younger. He made me feel the proudest I had felt in a long time. He'd not only made the decision to change, but the commitment to change. When I asked him what changes he'd made, it was simple. He had changed his habits. Now he didn't even want the foods he once craved.

Make the Change

People do make dramatic lifestyle changes so they don't have to go through an amputation like that man in the emergency room and wish they had made changes years earlier. Or they undergo a stent procedure that wakes them up to the need to do something.

Yet another reason people change is that they read and acquire wisdom about what they can do to prevent problems with their future health. In terms of motivation, that is the most challenging impetus for people to change, but it is the best one.

Gaining the knowledge for defeating diabetes and committing to do whatever it takes is the key. Developing proper habits prevents you from having to go through a complication of diabetes, an associated arterial problem with your heart or your brain, or a blockage in the large artery to your leg that forces you to undergo an amputation.

Make the commitment to change before you experience a medical problem. Understand what happens to thousands of diabetics who rely only on their medication to fight the disease. Realize the associated risk factors that affect your arteries to your heart, brain, and legs as well as to every organ of your body.

I hope this book will be your number one reason for changing your lifestyle habits. It would be great to know that you're learning what's going on in your body, plus what you can do to make a difference. Knowing that would make me feel fantastic, especially if I don't have to get a call from you at 5:42 in the morning.

How to Drop Bad Habits for Good Ones

Recently a lady who was obese told me she had to change her life because she was constantly miserable and going down a slippery slope. Her eating habits were terrible. She kept a bowl of candy on her desk for anyone to take a sample, but she ended up eating at least half of the supply herself. She was diabetic and on blood pressure medication, "but the medication isn't controlling my pressure very well," she said. She had *wanted* to lose weight and get on a healthy diet several times before, but she'd never been successful. Yet something inside her made her realize it was time to change, this time for good.

We are all like this lady, at least in some ways. We *want* to do so many things, but we just don't get organized enough to accomplish them.

Bad habits are difficult to change. It's hard to stop sitting on the couch watching television and form the habit of personal exercise five to six days a week. It's difficult to quit the eating habits that have made us overweight and instead develop the habits of proper eating.

I see many individuals who *want to* improve their health. Most everyone has that desire, but very few have the commitment to get it accomplished. Why is that? What does it take to finally realize you need to do something to change the dreaded road you're on? How do you change bad habits for good ones?

The problem is, desire is of the mind and requires no action. Commitment is of the heart and does require action. But the fact that you're reading this book says something inside you knows you want to change the direction of your life, and you're ready to commit.

I learned a secret years ago that answers how to change bad habits into good ones. It's a bit of wisdom that has stood the test of time for me. I hope it will do the same for you.

When I began the difficult road of medical school, I rented an apartment from Mrs. Avery. Her husband had died of a heart attack eight years prior, and since then she had surrounded herself with medical students. We were not yet physicians, but I assumed she felt safer with us there. The rent was cheap, the accommodations were clean, and best of all, my two roommates and I were left alone in quiet. I remember choosing the corner room with its big bed and a large antique desk. I assumed the desk was something out of Mr. Avery's insurance office.

The first night of studying my notes from that day's anatomy class, sitting at that desk, I noticed something written and underlined, most likely by Mr. Avery, in the upper right-hand corner of the old felt pad: *Set your goals high.* I remember thinking if I wanted to become a doctor, I was going to have to set some goals and commit to them. I had been accepted into medical school toward the end of the list because my grades weren't as good as many other applicants'. I knew I was at a point in my life where I had to make a decision that was going to determine the rest of my days.

I wrote on the felt pad too: *Major goal—become a doctor.* Underneath, I put: *Intermediate goal—make an A in Anatomy.* Below that I printed: *Immediate action goal— study every minute.*

I knew I was going to have to change the study habits I had in college. I enjoyed college by doing a lot of things other than studying. Sitting at that desk, I made the commitment to make my immediate action goal for that day to study every minute I was out of class except for eating. I studied that night until midnight. The next evening after dinner at the fraternity house, instead of playing a relaxing game of ping-pong or watching football previews on television, I went straight to my room and began studying, again until midnight. That weekend I drove to my future wife's parents' house and studied all Saturday afternoon. After dinner, I studied only until ten rather than twelve, but I had my commitment in order.

The commitment I made that first evening in medical school is the same commitment I want for you. The immediate action goal of making myself study as hard as I could that weekend was what determined whether I would become a doctor.

Once I set those goals, I never thought of changing them. No matter how bad the odds became, I never played with the idea. I believe that initial step of commitment is the reason I succeeded in becoming a physician. Studying became a habit.

I encourage you to make a similar decision about your desire to defeat your diabetes. Set it as a major goal, and never change it. Your intermediate goals may be anything from losing weight to exercising, but I remind you that your immediate action goal is the deciding factor. Your immediate action goal is what you're going to do about it today. At the end of today, you'll know whether you'll be successful in eating the proper foods, following your personal exercise program, and reaching your ideal weight because you'll know whether you've made the commitment.

Setting Goals for Success

Defeating diabetes presents many challenges. Each one must be identified and met with a plan. Your *major goal* is defeating diabetes. Depending on what other health risk factors you have, you will set several *intermediate goals* to accomplish. Your success will ultimately depend on how well you handle your *immediate action goals* on a day-to-day basis to develop the habits that will lead to success.

Every day you will choose whether you're going to exercise, whether you're going to take your "exercise medicine." You'll decide whether you're going to avoid a certain food. You'll take daily steps to reach your goal weight. Your main goal in weight loss is not losing the weight, but even more important, maintaining that goal weight number when you get there. I encourage you to set goals for what you want to accomplish.

Then write them down. If you write down what you plan to do, your goals are much more likely to be reached. Write down your goal weight on a sticky note and place it on your bathroom mirror. Write out your personal menu for each meal for a week. Write down when and where you're going to exercise each day and what that exercise will be and what clothes and running shoes you'll wear. Write down what you're going to do the next time you want a snack. (More about this soon, but detail what you'll do for the ten minutes after that snack desire hits you: what non-caloric drink you will consume, whom you will call, or what book you will pick up to read instead of eating that snack.)

I encourage you to give it a try. Write down your major goal and each intermediate goal you need to accomplish, as well as how you're going to react immediately today to accomplish the lifestyle habits you need to form.

Just remember, as I have learned, that writing them down is almost like magic.

The Significance of Desire

When do you plan to exchange bad health habits for good health habits? Will you wait for a major event like a heart attack, or being told you must be placed on insulin, or the first time your doctor starts you on high blood pressure medication, or when someone you know is just beginning to have symptoms of Alzheimer's?

With events like these, you'd probably at least consider changing your lifestyle habits. One example is the lady who teared up when she told me her doctor informed her she was diabetic and that the damage to her arteries was equivalent to having a first heart attack. Or the gentleman who wanted to know what to do because he had just had his first stent placed in an artery of his heart. He wanted to prevent ever having another one placed or ending up with a full-blown heart attack.

Both these people wanted to change their daily habits. Both realized they had to develop new habits that would make them healthier with a better quality of life. They both realized the way they had been living needed changing. The good news is you don't have to experience something bad before deciding to change your habits, but you do have to evaluate what habits you're going to need to change to successfully defeat your diabetes.

Most of what we do that's not good for us we do out of habit—making poor food choices, sitting on the couch watching television, buying the wrong foods, snacking too much. Habits are addictions. You fight those addictions by changing your habits to the point your good lifestyle choices become new habits. You start small with your changes, but the key is to beat the desire for a bad habit. Unless the desire is controlled, you'll eventually return to your old ways.

In most medical journal reports on weight loss, the follow-up numbers consistently show a 25 percent to 50 percent regain. People regain weight because desire wasn't beaten. Because foods can be addicting, you'll continue to desire certain foods unless you abstain from them completely for a certain period. The only way you can gain control of an addiction is by abstaining. You can develop the habit of not eating certain foods. Tomorrow you'll wholeheartedly avoid some of the foods you crave today because you'll realize what they've been doing to your health.

When I was rotating through orthopedic surgery during my surgical training program, the number two surgeon on the staff was in his forties and had smoked most of his life. He decided to quit smoking, and he enrolled in a program where he gradually cut down on the number of cigarettes he smoked every week. As time went on, he announced that he was down to three cigarettes a day. The next week he only smoked two per day, and finally the ultimate Friday came when he was to smoke his last cigarette.

We all gathered around and watched as he inhaled each draw. With his last puff, he tilted his head back and slowly blew out the smoke through his nostrils. He smashed the tip of the last cigarette into a small ashtray, and we all applauded and congratulated him. His smile was the biggest I had ever seen on him.

The problem was he had not beaten the desire for nicotine. The next Tuesday he lit another cigarette. By the end of the next week, he was back to smoking his routine pack a day.

Individuals have told me they were going to eat red meat only once a week. "Just on Saturday evenings," they would say. Or that they were going to eat dessert just once a week—as a reward for cutting out desserts. The problem is they retained the desire for the saturated fat or the sugary treat. The once-a-week plan never works permanently.

To lose weight and never regain it, you must beat the desire for the foods that put excess weight back on. It takes about two months, sixty days, of *abstaining*, for that desire to begin to fade. But once you reach that mark, it will become easier and easier to maintain that new habit you want to form. You take small steps to develop healthy habits, but you must defeat the desire factor as well, or you will never develop the right habits to defeat diabetes.

You not only have to beat the desires of your old habits, but you must replace them with desires for new good habits. With foods, it won't be enough to simply avoid that sugary dessert you have such a desire for now. You'll need to develop the habit of abstinence to the point you won't even want a single bite of it because you know what it will do to your health.

You will look at exercising the same way you look at taking medicine. If your doctor gives you a prescription for your health, you take it like clockwork. Look at exercise as taking medicine. Few people enjoy jogging or walking or most exercise routines, but when you realize how essential it is, you'll go through your exercise program the same way you take your medicine—routinely. Develop the habit of taking your "exercise medicine" five to six days a week. Before long, you will do it out of habit. You'll begin to react automatically to your new eating plan and exercise routines.

To change your lifestyle to one that can control your blood sugar, lose any excess weight, maintain the loss, and develop an exercise program, you will have to make some changes in your life. Some people will have many bad habits to replace with new ones. Others will need to only fine-tune what they're already doing. Whichever group you fit into, you can develop systems you can rely on automatically. You can't go through the rest of your life making decisions about which food you're going to avoid at each meal or whether you're going to exercise. Instead, you'll practice eating the right foods and exercising regularly out of habit.

Habits control our lives, so begin changing any bad habits you have to good habits today.

Habits to Live By

A habit is an unwritten rule. We follow them every day of our lives without thinking about them. We do them automatically, and if we don't make decisions and commitments to change them, we're going to aimlessly float down the river of life as it naturally flows.

If you're in that diabetic river, you can't afford to drift along. Steer your boat in the proper direction. If you don't make new rules for yourself, the old rules will lead to more problems, like high blood pressure, high cholesterol, a heart attack, or a stroke—not to mention eye problems and kidney difficulties or Alzheimer's.

Develop the right eating habits. Period. You don't want to have to decide whether to eat right every time you sit down to eat. You don't want to have to think twice. Eat a certain breakfast every day, out of habit. Eat certain lunches, out of habit. And for dinner, you may decide between three or four choices, but they will all be healthy and habitual. You will eat based on your new habits. If you form the right eating habits while you're losing weight, when you get to your ideal weight, you won't have to change a thing. Even better, you'll maintain that goal weight the rest of your life—*out of habit*. It works the same way with exercise. Exercise will become routine.

One morning I called a friend who had been overweight at one time and had developed the habit of exercising five days a week. When he answered the phone, he told me he was at the airport headed overseas for five days. He had risen early to get in his exercise on the treadmill and had his running gear packed so he wouldn't miss any days of exercise. Exercise became his habit the same way you will create eating and exercise habits to defeat your diabetes.

Every physician has explained to overweight diabetics what steps need to be taken to get to a proper weight. Sometimes we realize we're wasting our time as well as the diabetics' because they don't have the *desire* to change. If you're reading this book, you've already proven you have the desire to change. But there's much more to making changes than simply the desire to change. I'll say it again: Desire is of the mind and requires no action. Commitment is of the heart and does require action.

A significant part of your defeating diabetes will center on two major factors beyond the foods you eat: weight loss and exercise. I know you have the desire to lose the weight and to exercise, and when you commit to attacking weight loss and exercising, the odds are in your favor to defeat diabetes.

Willpower is a good initial step for something you desire to do, but unless you transform willpower into new habits, you'll eventually fall back into your old habits. Willpower usually lasts only from that last cigarette smoked on Friday until the following Tuesday, when your desire overcomes your willpower to the point of smoking a whole pack.

Beat the desire.

Triggers for Making Change

Being overweight is the number one factor to address as a diabetic. As I mentioned before, over 80 percent of diabetics fit into this category. I have talked to numerous individuals about losing weight. Some honestly desire to lose weight because something has happened to make them ready to commit to change. Others "want to" lose weight, but because a special event is coming up this next weekend, they assure me they will start first thing Monday morning. (I don't say anything to them, but the thought that runs through my mind is *tell that to your mother; she might believe you.*)

I read an article that said people who have succeeded in losing weight and keeping it off made the commitment to do so from the beginning. A study reported on in the *American Journal of Clinical Nutrition* tied the success to a "triggering event" that almost forced the individual to decide they were going to lose their excess weight. This study consisted of people who had been successful in losing their excess weight and able to maintain the weight loss for at least a year. Eighty-three percent of them reported a trigger event that began their weight loss, and that event was the encouraging factor that allowed them to continue permanently on that lifestyle of better eating and more exercise.

It's interesting to see what those triggers were. The most commonly reported event was a medical mishap. The next most common trigger was an individual realizing they had reached an all-time high in weight. The third most common trigger was looking at a picture of themselves or looking in the mirror and realizing how they looked.

One of these triggers made them decide they had to make a change, and that trigger continually lingered in their minds for years to come. The medical mishap triggers were having a heart attack or seeing someone in the family have one. Or having a stent placed in one of the arteries of their heart. Or a doctor telling the person what was going to happen if they didn't lose their excess weight. In this report, they found the people who had the medical triggers were more successful in losing weight and maintaining that weight loss than those who'd had any of the other triggers. Their conclusion reminds us that "the period following a medical trigger may be an opportune time to initiate weight loss to optimize both initial and long-term weight loss outcomes."

Sometimes people do need a jolt, like a heart attack or being told they have diabetes or high blood pressure or seeing a loved one show the first signs of Alzheimer's. Others can learn from reading about what's going to happen unless changes are made. My mother had a favorite expression she taught us boys. She said we didn't have to wait until something bad happened to us before making the decision to change our ways and do right. She wanted us to learn from her wisdom rather than waiting for something bad to happen before we decided to avoid the bad and do the good. My mother reminded us many times: "experience is a dear teacher—fools learn by no other."

Often, a time of crisis is the beginning of a downhill spiral, the first domino that causes the second and third to tumble. The initial domino may be your diabetes, but the second is high blood pressure, and then a third is a stent placed in an artery of your heart, followed by a full-blown heart attack or stroke. This is the tumbling effect. I don't know where you presently stand, but if a medical crisis has occurred, you must consider what is to come unless you begin taking preventive action. If you have had any of the above triggers, you should commit to change immediately.

But if you have not had to experience any of the above, I want this book to become a trigger, without having to physically go through such a disaster.

The biggest compliment I could ever get would be being told this book has taken the place of a medical trigger. Don't wait until you have that first heart attack. Don't wait on being told in the emergency room that you're going to have to have a stent placed in an artery in your heart. When you look in the mirror, you're looking at a person who can change your life. You don't have to stay on the road you're on.

You can begin today by believing in yourself. Believe you can lose weight. Believe you can get moving. Believe you can change your eating habits and form new ones. Believe it can happen.

9. Exercise

Excess weight is the number one culprit of diabetes, and that's why beginning an exercise program is your first step in defeating diabetes. Exercise is the habit that changes everything. It's extremely difficult to lose weight unless you do it. Losing excess weight and eating the right foods are both important, but if you don't exercise, your battle is going to be tough.

Exercise is much more than burning a certain number of calories. Your body uses about a hundred calories per mile, whether you're walking or running. If you compare overweight diabetics who exercise to those who don't, you'll see the ones who exercise also do significantly better with their eating and lose a lot more weight.

I like to cite a Brown University study that compared two groups of overweight women. One group dieted and exercised while the other group only dieted. The group that dieted *and* exercised lost almost *twice* the weight ones who didn't exercise lost. Those numbers make a clear statement about the significance of exercise. If you want to lose weight and keep it off, do more than just diet.

Exercise is also the one best lifestyle change that will inspire your confidence in succeeding. It's the one *immediate action* behavior that will give you the self-assurance that you can tackle and master other necessary lifestyle changes. Small, habitual changes will eventually lead to permanent healthy lifestyle changes that will defeat your diabetes as well as prevent the heart trouble, high blood pressure problems, LDL cholesterol complications, and Alzheimer's diabetes is leading you toward.

If you're overweight, you'll address weight loss by eating properly, but you want your plan to be successful in maintaining weight loss as well as losing the weight. That's why medical reports that study the individuals who have successfully lost the weight and kept it off are so helpful.

What Medical Studies Tell Us about Exercise

The ongoing study that shows this reality best is conducted by the National Weight Control Registry. They're following participants who have lost an average of sixty-six pounds and kept it off an average of five and a half years. These individuals are good examples for all of us to follow. Of the participants in this study, 90 percent exercised, on average, about one hour per day. Let's look at an article published in *Journal of Physical Activity and Health* concerning these successful weight-loss individuals. The study compared the ones who did the most exercise with the ones who did a low amount of exercise.

This study looked at the intensity of the activity being high versus low, but keep in mind that even the lowest intensity of exercise is great for a diabetic. Don't be discouraged if your exercise plan initially includes only walking.

The study showed that those participants who exercised the most were not only more likely to lose more weight and maintain the loss than those who exercised the least, but were more likely to take many other positive actions that affected their weight. Researchers found the participants who were the most serious about their exercise routine also followed their proper eating lifestyle better.

This is the most important lesson concerning exercise and weight loss and maintaining your new weight. Exercise enhances your determination to also improve other lifestyle choices. If you exercise every day on schedule, you're much more likely to do all the other things that go along with losing weight and controlling your diabetes.

Remember, many factors are intertwined with having diabetes. Diabetes is an arterial risk factor. That means it falls into the same category as other health problems that affect the health of your arteries that can result in a heart attack or stroke or Alzheimer's. All these risk factors are inter-reactive. Having one of the risks increases your odds of having another. The diabetic risk factor for the health of your arteries increases your odds of being overweight. Being overweight increases your odds of having high blood pressure. Most diabetics don't exercise, which plays a role in their cholesterol. They're all intertwined and must be addressed together.

Exercise is a key to success in other areas that make an impact not only on your diabetes but on your overall health. Many studies have revealed that the participants who exercised the most not only followed their proper eating routines better, but also lost higher levels of weight and achieved the lowest overall body weight. The higher level of physical activity resulted in greater weight loss and a more consistent maintenance. The physically active participants reported more extreme behaviors concerning other factors that ensured weight-loss maintenance. Not only did they engage in more dietary weight control behaviors, but they also had a lower intake of saturated fatty foods and refrained from eating unhealthy foods.

Defeating diabetes means taking on several issues. Yes, being overweight is the worst of the worst, but many other factors must be addressed. Exercise plays a huge role in going into a successful battle against diabetes, and I encourage you to begin if you haven't started, and to persist if you have. Exercising consistently makes you more likely to do the other things necessary to win the battle.

A report in *Journal of Internal Medicine* shows the impact of exercise on mortality. After a follow-up of diabetics who exercised and diabetics who didn't, their concluding statement was this: "Amongst confirmed diabetic persons, increased physical activity is associated with significant decrease of mortality."

Exercise Is Essential

The *Cleveland Clinic Journal of Medicine* published an article highlighting several key points on the importance of exercise for diabetics. The article states that "exercise is an essential component of all diabetes and obesity prevention and lifestyle intervention programs." Also, that "exercise is central to effective lifestyle prevention and management of type 2 diabetes."

I wholeheartedly agree with their comment that the combination of aerobic and resistance training, as recommended by current American Diabetic Association guidelines, may be the most effective exercise modality for controlling glucose and fats in type 2 diabetes. The authors explain that, following a meal, your skeletal muscle is the primary site for glucose disposal and uptake. Much of the insulin resistance originates in these muscles and is a major driver for the development of type 2 diabetes. Exercise enhances the uptake of glucose by these muscles and results in improved sensitivity to insulin being able to let the glucose through the door into the muscle cells.

The bottom line of this report is that individuals who maintain a physically active lifestyle can reduce their risk of developing type 2 diabetes as well as improve their heart profile. Diabetics are two to four times more likely than healthy individuals to suffer from heart disease, resulting in a heart attack or heart failure. Exercise can improve both entities at the same time. Such reports are a strong indication that exercise does more than just burn a certain number of calories.

Exercise and Ideal Weight

Which is more important—exercise or ideal weight? The answer is both.

An article in *Diabetes Care* reviews several trials that focused on medication as compared to lifestyle changes. These numbers show why lifestyle changes can be *better* than medication, and also why it's important to maintain your weight loss once you've achieved it. These studies show a 58 percent reduction in prediabetic patients progressing to being diagnosed as diabetic when they changed their lifestyles, including beginning to exercise. That percentage, however, dropped to 43 percent at seven years and 34 percent at ten years because the weight-loss participants achieved the first year wasn't maintained. These studies demonstrate the importance exercise plays in maintaining weight loss.

An article in the *New England Journal of Medicine* reinforces the significance one lifestyle choice plays on the next. All three lifestyle choices are intertwined and equally important. This report substantiates that obesity and physical inactivity are the two main determining factors of diabetes. Researchers ran a trial on 522 middle-aged overweight adults who had impaired glucose tolerance. Their glucose was elevated, but not to the extent of being diagnosed as diabetic. They were divided into two groups. One group was given some instructions on weight loss, but the other group underwent exercise profiling and were given specifics for their diet, consisting of decreasing their intake of saturated fat as well as increasing their intake of fiber. Their exercise consisted mainly of walking. The group that ate properly and exercised had a 58 percent less incidence of developing diabetes. Studies on prediabetics are equally relevant to diabetics. With both categories, you are studying how to fight elevated blood sugar no matter what degree that elevation happens to be.

A key point to take away is that the more you exercise, the better, but in this study, we learn even simple walking produced huge gains in reducing the chance of developing diabetes. Just remember, even a slow walk fifteen minutes a day five or six days a week is significant. I say this because before long, you will be doing a thirty-minute slow walk per day, and that will turn into a brisk walk. Down the road you may surprise yourself into trotting some of the time and then perhaps jogging. The main point is to begin a personal exercise program.

Years ago, an overweight friend decided he wanted to begin exercising. He knew I ran three miles a day, so he asked if he could join me. The road I ran beside was paved but out of town with very little traffic. We started at a bridge. I told him where the mile-and-a-half marker was, that I ran there and back, and that he should keep running but turn around when he saw me coming back. About a quarter of a mile down the road was the first mailbox. He wasn't much past that mailbox as I was finishing my run. He had jogged to the mailbox and then walked the remaining time. But in a month's time, he was doing a slow jog for thirty minutes each day.

Don't get discouraged. Set your goal, and at least walk briskly to that first mailbox. If you do that and stick with it, you can defeat the two main culprits of diabetes: being overweight and inactive.

Walking Is Exercise

Committing to an exercise routine five to six days a week is paramount. What you do for your routine is a personal choice, whether walking four blocks or running a four-minute mile. But an excellent article published in the *Archives of Internal Medicine* addresses the importance of walking for all diabetics.

It begins with a statement that shouldn't surprise you: "Physical inactivity is a major cause of type 2 diabetes mellitus, and increasing physical activity level is associated with substantial reduction in the risk of type 2 diabetes." The study concludes that brisk walking for at least thirty minutes a day is associated with a 30 to 40 percent reduction in risk of type 2 diabetes. For those who have prediabetes, such exercise can prevent most cases of diabetes. Those already diagnosed as diabetic can achieve a similar effect. Researchers compared diabetics who performed walking exercise with those taking the popular medication—metformin—and found lifestyle modification was a far more effective therapy for their diabetes than the medicine.

As a diabetic, you have an increased risk of heart failure and heart attacks. Think of the quality of the years you have left to live. The above article reports that regular walking of a half hour per day was associated with an approximately 50 percent lower risk of heart attack and total mortality in a group of 2,896 adults with diabetes. The chance to cut my risk of dying from a heart attack by 50 percent would make me consistently take my "exercise medicine."

The article also reviewed other studies where diabetic patients who were being treated for their cholesterol or high blood pressure—on statins, insulin, and oral medications for their diabetes—had better benefits with a moderate amount of walking than they had with medications for treating the disorders mentioned above.

The compelling results of these studies show the benefits of exercising. The report above focused on walking briskly. It also included a study showing that seven hours a week of moderate to vigorous exercise was associated with a greater reduction in the incidence of heart attacks. That means the more strenuous the exercise, the better odds of protection you will have.

The point to remember is that simple walking improves your health and protects you against the number one cause of death in diabetics. Walking thirty minutes a day is a thousandfold better than sitting on the couch. Walking is an exercise that most everyone can do, even if overweight or elderly. I like the researchers' concluding statement: "Walking is probably the 'best medicine' for both prevention and treatment of diabetes mellitus."

An Exercise Plan That Works for You

It doesn't matter whether you presently exercise a lot or not at all. The objective is to either get started or fine-tune your exercise program to make sure you're getting your heart rate elevated for a continuous thirty minutes a day. Remember, exercise addresses your diabetes as well as strengthens your heart.

The following exercise plan is going to work for you, whether you're a couch potato or already exercise every day. We want to strengthen the heart muscle, and exercise is the only thing that does that. No medicine will do it. Strengthening your heart muscle is similar to strengthening your biceps. The more you exercise it, the thicker and stronger the heart muscle gets. If you put a work force on the muscle, it responds by getting stronger. The more work force you place on your heart, the more times it will beat per minute during that work force.

To see the advantage of exercise, we look at a report in the journal *Archives of Internal Medicine*, which showed that jogging was linked with an added 6.2 years to the life expectancies for men and 5.6 years to the life expectancies for women.

If you have diabetes and add exercise to your schedule, you will see your weight decrease along with improvement in your diabetes numbers. Remember the Brown University study that had the entire group on the same weight loss diet but half of them exercised and half didn't. The half that exercised lost almost twice the weight as the ones who didn't exercise.

The most significant reason exercise such as jogging extends your life is that it strengthens your heart muscle. The reasoning goes like this: the best exercise you can do to strengthen your heart is to sustain a significantly high heart rate for a thirty-minute interval. Multiple trials show that maximum strength of your heart muscle is obtained by keeping the heart rate above the 80th percentile of your maximum rate during that interval. To figure your personal 80th percentile rate, subtract your age from the number 220. That gives you your maximum heart rate. Eighty percent of that number is your goal rate to achieve.

Such heart-strengthening exercise can be accomplished even with brisk walking. In the plan being presented, that brisk walking can be slowly increased to the point of jogging. Aerobic exercise not only strengthens your heart muscle but also helps you lose weight and fight diabetes.

Set thirty minutes a day as your aerobic exercise period, whether you're walking or jogging. If you haven't jogged before, begin with a brisk walk for thirty minutes a day. No matter where you are on the fitness continuum, the important word is *begin*. Your walk can be done on a track or a treadmill or a path, and then slowly increase your pace over several weeks. If you can't jog yet, begin with a thirty-minute walk every day at a steady pace for a one-week period. Once you feel comfortable with your thirty-minute brisk walk, begin adding a two-minute jog at the beginning of the brisk walk routine. Then add another two minutes a week to the beginning of your brisk walk routine and gradually increase your jogging time until you're doing a full thirty-minute jog five to six days a week. All the while, your heart is getting stronger and stronger.

Here is a good self-test to determine if you're exercising enough to get your heart muscle working at peak performance. You can do it after you finish your brisk walk or fast jog, or whatever you're doing that gets your heart rate above the 80th percentile. After finishing your thirty minutes, count your pulse at the end of one minute and again at the end of two minutes. As your heart muscle gets toward optimum strength, your pulse rate will drop more and more dramatically just after completing your exercise. You will know your heart muscle is at its peak performance when you find that your rate drops twenty-five beats by the end of the first minute after completing your aerobic exercise and drops an additional fifteen beats by the end of your second minute.

Committing to a thirty-minute walk may be the most significant decision you'll make in this journey. You will have "begun."

Have I encouraged you enough? Not every diabetic can run a four-minute mile, but the overwhelming majority can walk. The commitment to exercise is far more beneficial than sitting on the sofa.

The Effect of Exercise on Insulin Resistance in Diabetics

Why does exercise have such an important effect on diabetes? The answer relates to insulin resistance. You recall the role of insulin resistance in the overall diabetes problem. Exercise plays a significant role in making cells switch from being insulin resistant to becoming insulin sensitive.

A study published in *Journal of Clinical Endocrinologic Metabolism* divided type 2 diabetics into two groups, with both groups dieting and one group doing both diet and exercise. The group that dieted and exercised had a greater improvement in decrease in body fat and BMI as well as an increase in insulin sensitivity. The significant point was that insulin sensitivity was greatly increased with exercise. The study measured the rate of infusion of insulin into muscle cells, and the participants who exercised had a 57 percent increase in uptake of glucose from the blood into the cells.

If You're Diabetic, Will You Die Sooner If You Don't Exercise?

All these reports show good results with exercise as it relates to both diabetes and heart health. But what about mortality? Does exercise really help determine if you're going to die before you should, even if you have diabetes? That's a good question, and you're about to read the answer.

In a study published in the journal *Diabetes Care*, 2,196 diabetic men were followed for an average of over fourteen years. They were placed into one of three groups, according to how much they exercised. They found the risk of mortality was inversely related to fitness in a steep gradient between degrees of exercise performed. The better physical condition, the lower the mortality rate. The study concluded that the ones who exercised the least had a greater than five times higher risk of death than those who exercised the most.

Another article in the *Archives of Internal Medicine* makes it even plainer. The study it discussed noted a significantly higher risk of heart attack if a person is diabetic than if not.

This article stressed that physical activity is the cornerstone of managing diabetes. Researchers based this on the fact that persons with diabetes are at higher risk for disease of the arteries of their heart and brain and are subject to premature death. The study recommended at least 150 minutes per week of moderate-intensity aerobic physical activity, with walking being of particular interest because it requires no specific facilities and can be easily performed in a daily routine and is relatively safe. The study concludes, "Physical activity relates to a thirty-three percent lower risk of overall mortality and a thirty-five percent lower risk of heart mortality compared with inactivity."

You don't have to be a doctor to understand the reward of exercise if you're diabetic. And remember, we're not just talking about how long you will live but also about quality of life. Living longer isn't rewarding if your quality of life is greatly impaired. Think of your new lifestyle changes in terms of not only getting to live longer but also living life with more quality.

More about Exercise and Mortality

We rightly give much attention to the care of blood glucose in diabetics. Diet is important, and control of the level of glucose in the blood is paramount in not letting it get too high or too low. Entire books have been written on controlling glucose levels throughout the day and night. One significant article published in the *Annals of Internal Medicine* looks at the factors that determine whether you will die earlier than you should and what can be done to postpone an early mortality if you're diabetic. To me, these are practical studies we want to know about. *Winning Your Blood Sugar Battle* is about more than how much medicine you take to regulate your glucose. This study compares your "prescribed medicine" with your "lifestyle medicine" as related to your heart. Which is more important?

The study consisted of over twelve hundred men who had type 2 diabetes and were followed for 11.7 years. They were categorized into three groups, according to how much they exercised—low fit, moderate fit, and high fit. This was based on what percent heart rate they achieved during their exercise periods.

The greater the exercise, the more protective effect. The study found that exercise not only helped in overweight individuals but also helped in diabetics who were not overweight. Exercise didn't just help patients lose weight; it helped in glucose control, in lowered blood pressure, and in improving their cholesterol profile and increasing their sensitivity to insulin. All this resulted in improved mortality rates. The ones who were in the lowest exercise profile had increased rates of death from cardiac disease leading to heart attacks.

These researchers concluded that thirty minutes a day of moderate-intensity exercise such as brisk walking is sufficient to develop and maintain the fitness level associated with the lower mortality rates found in their study.

Exercise will improve your glucose, but it will also improve your cholesterol numbers, lower your blood pressure, decrease your weight, and lower your risk of a heart attack or stroke. That is a lot to say in one sentence, but I will show you some medical reports that affirm these results.

More Studies about the Effects of Exercise

An article in the *New England Journal of Medicine* reported on the reduction of occurrence of diabetes with exercise. Researchers pointed out that active exercise not considered extreme—such as jogging at five miles per hour, bicycling at a rapid pace, or swimming laps at a moderate pace—were significantly effective in decreasing diabetes. Yet less intense exercise also had a significant effect. They listed exercise as one of the main factors, along with diet and weight control, effective in defeating diabetes.

Another study published in the *British Medical Journal* produced similar results. Intensive exercise improved insulin sensitivity 58 to 98 percent in their study of 129 obese patients with diabetes. It also improved their A1c, blood pressure, LDL cholesterol, and HDL cholesterol. An extra parameter included in the study was the significance of weight loss, with exercise resulting in a 25 percent reduction of mortality with such loss.

Such studies continue to reiterate that exercise addresses two crucial issues for diabetics: glucose control and the health of the heart. Exercise improves the sensitivity of your cells to insulin and at the same time improves the health of your heart.

An article published in the *Journal of the American Medical Association* puts it all into proper perspective. This study showed the coexistence of type 2 diabetes and high blood pressure, causing significant damage to the heart of diabetics.

Having high blood pressure is bad for anyone, but it's even more damaging to the arteries of the heart for diabetics. This report stated that some studies showed "a prevalence of high blood pressure being associated as high as sixty percent in persons with type 2 diabetes." The article emphasized that most diabetics die of complication problems of the arteries of the heart and brain resulting in heart attacks and stroke. This statement is significant: "Having type 2 diabetes increases the risk of cardiovascular disease two to four-fold." Another astonishing result was the increased risk of having an event in the heart if you have diabetes and high blood pressure, compared to people who aren't diabetic: "Some data estimate a doubling of cardiovascular events when hypertension and diabetes coexist."

Not only does this article point out the dangers of the coexistence of high blood pressure and excess weight for diabetics, but it tells what can be done to combat them. It emphasizes that exercise is a "major therapeutic modality for type 2 diabetes," stating that the American Diabetes Association says that "the possible benefits of exercise in type 2 diabetes are substantial, and the American College of Sports Medicine says that physical activity is a major therapeutic modality for type 2 diabetes."

All these groups are telling how important it is for you to exercise if you're diabetic. That is why exercise is given first place for you to begin to change your lifestyle.

Not only has aerobic exercise been shown to be beneficial, but also resistance training, where multiple muscle groups of the body are exercised. *Diabetes Care* published a study that showed that weight loss alone increases insulin sensitivity and exercise alone increases it, but exercise and weight loss together have an even greater effect on insulin sensitivity. Their study on insulin sensitivity in relation to resistance exercise showed that insulin sensitivity increased by 46 percent. There was no conclusion as to exactly how working our muscle masses improves insulin sensitivity, but researchers speculated that it may be related to exercise increasing glucose storage areas in the muscle. This could facilitate the clearance of glucose from the circulation and reduce the amount of insulin required to maintain a normal glucose level. This study was based on the participants lifting weights and performing muscle resistance exercise twice a week. This may be an encouragement to do such exercises two days a week in addition to the cardio exercise.

In Conclusion

As we conclude this discussion of the importance of exercise for diabetics, this quote from an article published in the *Annals of Internal Medicine* puts it all in proper perspective: "Cardiovascular disease is the leading cause of death in persons with diabetes mellitus." Researchers conducted a fourteen-year study of diabetics and found how the health of their arteries affected mortality. Disease of the heart arteries, resulting in heart attacks, accounted for 50 percent of the deaths, and disease of the arteries in the brain, causing strokes, accounted for an additional 15 percent of deaths.

Their study evaluated the effect of exercise on both heart attacks and strokes over a fourteen-year follow-up. They compared individuals who exercised less than one hour a week with those who exercised more than seven hours a week. The most common exercise was brisk walking. The ones who exercised seven hours per week were twice as likely to not have a heart attack or stroke. Even the ones who spent at least four hours per week performing moderate or vigorous exercise had an approximately 40 percent lower risk of a heart attack or stroke. Researchers concluded that levels of physical activity were inversely associated with heart artery disease causing both heart attacks and stroke. The more the diabetics exercised, the less chance they had of having a heart attack or stroke.

This report showed that exercise has beneficial effect on your glucose control, as well as improving your insulin resistance, reducing your weight, and improving your cholesterol profile. In this study, exercise improved their "hero" HDL cholesterol by 25 percent. It's good to know all the things you're improving as you take your brisk walk each day.

I like the study's conclusion about even moderate exercise among diabetics: "Our study provides strong evidence that regular walking, especially brisk walking, is associated with lower risk for coronary heart disease and stroke."

Multiple studies reinforce the conclusion that regular exercise is the key to developing the quality of life you want. Quality of life comes with a price, but it's worth every exercise step you take to attain it. Exercise is the best medicine you can take if you're diabetic. You take your other medicine, so take your "exercise medicine" as well.

10. What Should You Eat?

In this chapter you'll see an emphasis on some of what we've already touched on. For instance, you'll read more about red meat, eggs, and nuts. But, again, I want to be sure you have all the benefit of recent research as you make the commitment to change your lifestyle choices, including what you eat, as well as some tools to help make the best food choices.

I recently visited a hospital in a primitive area of New Guinea. The capital city was like many of the larger cities in America. They were building a new Hilton hotel and had several skyscrapers, and the people who lived and worked there made a good living. But out in the countryside, life was different.

One Sunday we drove to a little church two miles out on a dirt road. Passing one little village after another, I was informed that the people lived off the land, eating primarily what they grew in their gardens. Some had a pig or two, but they didn't eat them because that livestock was like a bank account. If an emergency came up, they could sell a pig to get the money they needed.

I asked the doctors at the mission hospital if they had many diabetics. Their response was that heart attacks and diabetes were seldom seen fifteen years ago, but now that the smaller towns were becoming more westernized, they were beginning to see more of those medical problems.

"When all they had to eat were the vegetables out of their garden, we didn't see diabetes or heart attacks. But now a typical lunch a worker buys in town consists of a soda and three or four flour balls."

When he explained what a flour ball was, I understood why they were beginning to treat more diabetics. To make a flour ball, people took a handful of flour, added a scoop of butter, mixed it all together, and then dropped it into a pot of grease and fried it. Three of them, along with a sugary soda, would fill them up for the day. The weight of the people who became "westernized" began to increase, and as the economy improved, the diet changed. What one eats definitely plays a role in diabetes.

That's a good example of how not to eat to defeat diabetes, but the question remains, What *should* someone with diabetes eat?

Although several diets for diabetics are out there, not one represents a conclusive approach. Some say to eat as few carbohydrates as possible because the carbs cause the glucose to be high and require extra insulin. Others say it's not the carbohydrates, but the high-glycemic carb foods that break down quickly and cause a spike in blood sugar. Some say you should carry with you some foods with extra sugar to eat in case your sugar gets low during the day. Others say never take in extra sugar; lower your insulin dose instead.

Multiple approaches to losing weight also exist. Some say rather than eating three meals a day, eat small amounts of food throughout the day. Some advise eating a low-carbohydrate/high-fat diet, while others *emphasize* a high-fat diet. Hopefully, this chapter will help clear up some of the confusion about what foods you should eat to lose weight, but whatever diet you adopt, look for foods that have fewer calories while also keeping you from being hungry all the time.

It's confusing when some people say a high-fat diet is better but others maintain that a high-carbohydrate diet is better. Both are wrong, and both are right! The reason is because there are both good fats and bad fats and both good carbs and bad carbs.

People who advocate a high-fat/low-carbohydrate diet don't distinguish between good fat and bad; they just say to eat fat instead of carbs. A diabetic once explained to me how she followed this plan. Her normal breakfast included two eggs with bacon or ham. Because of her medication, she was even able to include biscuits and gravy on occasion, but she stayed mainly with the high fat in the bacon and ham.

Her diet was low in carbohydrates, but here's the problem: it didn't address foods that affect the arteries of the heart and brain. Never forget the associated risks you have if you're diabetic. Everyone with diabetes has a significant increase in the risk of death or health problems related to the health of the arteries in their heart. Don't address one problem and ignore the other risk factors. The low-carb/high-protein diet may keep your glucose low, but it's playing havoc with your arteries in the meantime.

Other people maintain that eating carbohydrates is a good approach, but they caution you to focus on the type of carbohydrates you eat. They say to avoid the refined sugars found in sodas and sweets like cakes and donuts, and to eat a diet consisting of the carbohydrates found in high-fiber foods, like many vegetables and fruits and whole grains. Carbs higher in fiber are released slowly and digested without the spikes in glucose, which require your body to produce large amounts of insulin quickly.

To make this simple for you, let me put it this way: *avoid the bad fats and eat the good fats instead.* The same with carbohydrates: *avoid the bad carbohydrates and eat the good carbohydrates instead.* The fats bad for your arteries are the saturated fats found in red meat, cheese, egg yolk, butter, cream, and most fried foods. The good fats are found in fish, nuts, olive oil, and avocados. Good carbohydrates are high in fiber, like those found in vegetables, whole grains, and fruit. Of course, the refined sugars are the bad carbs found in things like desserts and packaged sweets.

Just remember this the next time you hear the two diets debated: it's about good and bad fats and good and bad carbs. Keep this in mind and develop your eating plan around both. By doing so, you can develop a plan that both controls your glucose level and protects the arteries of your heart and brain.

Everyone is different, and that's why I recommend working out your personal eating plan with your doctor. You will need to balance the glucose in the foods you eat with the number of medications you take and the timing of them. When you understand how your body handles different foods, you can understand what you should eat and what you should avoid.

Changing your diet involves more than learning how to keep your insulin in check. If we back up a step and learn how to address the two main risk factors associated with diabetes, then you'll find controlling your insulin level much simpler. Learning how to protect your heart with lifestyle changes gives you a double bonus.

The Most Nutritious Foods with the Fewest Calories

What you eat doesn't affect only your glucose and arteries; it also plays a role with your weight. Your weight-loss eating habits boil down to one issue: calories. Whatever diet you follow, the number of calories you take in must be fewer than the calories you burn. It doesn't matter what foods you eat or how much food you eat, if you put more calories into your system than your body uses, you will not lose weight.

The key is knowing which foods provide the most nutrition with the fewest calories. Keep in mind both the effect of the foods on your blood sugar and their effect on your arteries. This is not an either/or diet. Develop eating habits that protect your glucose level and your heart.

What are the best foods to fill you up with the least number of calories, so you won't feel hungry long before your next meal? The answer is vegetables, fruits, and beans. That's why it's so important to make salad a major part of your eating habits. A salad alone or with a small portion of fruit or beans or grilled chicken or fish added can fill your stomach. That makes a great lunch, and you can get all the vegetables you need by beginning your evening meal with a salad and variety of vegetables.

Is Red Meat Really Bad for You?

An article in *American Journal of Clinical Nutrition* presents a good study on whether red meat consumption is associated with increasing the risk of type 2 diabetes. The beginning of the report emphasizes what we've been discussing, pointing out that "although obesity and physical inactivity are major determinants of type 2 diabetes . . . dietary factors also play an important role in its development."

So what about red meat?

The researchers examined the effect of eating certain foods other than red meat. When comparing one serving of red meat per day to one serving of nuts, they found an associated 21 percent lower risk of type 2 diabetes among the participants who ate the nuts.

When comparing one serving of red meat per day to a serving of whole grain, there was a 23 percent lower risk of type 2 diabetes in those who ate the whole grain.

Poultry and fish each showed a 10 percent lower risk over red meat.

Researchers even broke it down into unprocessed red meat as well as processed meats, such as sausage or hot dogs, and found that both processed and unprocessed red meat are associated with a higher risk of diabetes. They noted that eating red meat is positively associated with a future risk of weight gain.

No risk stands alone. Being diabetic carries a number of factors you can control. Eating red meat is connected with becoming overweight, and that's associated with increasing your odds of having high blood pressure. As you read studies like these, notice that the various risk factors relate to lifestyle choices you can change.

Why would red meat be bad for a diabetic? Remember, we keep two things in mind: glucose and the heart. Saturated fat is strongly associated with red meats. And as you will recall, saturated fat is the one bad fat we eat the most of in America, which causes a rise in LDL cholesterol. LDL cholesterol is a primary cause of inflammation and plaque buildup in our arteries. Saturated fat stimulates the liver to produce more LDL cholesterol splinters. Therefore, don't eat the saturated fat. Avoid it. Don't eat it even in moderation; just avoid it. Don't eat red meat, cheese, egg yolk, butter, cream, and fried foods.

Don't focus only on the sugar you eat; think also about the fat. I sometimes wonder why God didn't place pain fibers in the walls of our arteries. I know it's far-fetched, but I also know we wouldn't eat the bad fatty foods that cause LDL splinters if we experienced pain every time we ate a bite of bad fat. Can you imagine how your diet would change if every time you ate red meat, you began feeling splinters all through your body? I suspect you would never eat that food again.

Unfortunately, we don't experience pain with every bite of bad food. But down the road, we might have the pain of a diabetic foot problem, or experience the pain associated with heart attack symptoms, or know the numbness and tingling pain of a developing stroke.

Since you don't experience immediate pain when you eat the wrong foods, let me draw a mental picture to remind you what can happen down the road if you continue to consume a lot of saturated fat.

The Carbohydrate Factor

Different types of carbohydrates are processed by the body in different ways. Some carbs are immediately absorbed with a resulting spike in the blood glucose level. This requires an immediate supply of insulin to help get the glucose out of the blood and into the cells. As you recall, with diabetes you have a resistance to insulin, and even if your pancreas increases the amount of insulin needed, the insulin key can't unlock the cell's door to let the extra glucose in.

The foods immediately absorbed are called foods with a *high glycemic index*, meaning they are quickly broken down and absorbed, resulting in that spike in blood sugar. These foods are often called "white foods," and include food like white bread, baked goods, juices, baked potatoes, and white rice.

The Fiber Factor

Fiber plays an important role in the foods we all choose, but particularly for diabetics. You should eat a diet high in the kinds of carbohydrates that don't cause a flush effect on your blood glucose after a meal. High fiber content helps control your blood sugar level. Choose foods that have the highest nutrition with the fewest calories that don't flood your bloodstream with an abundance of glucose. As previously mentioned, fiber content in a food is digested differently and releases glucose into your system much more slowly.

The carbohydrate in fiber is compacted so tightly that it's digested much more slowly or not at all.

Different foods have different amounts of fiber. Many vegetables and fruits contain the fiber that protects you against glucose surges. Begin focusing on vegetables and beans as mainstays. You don't have to become a vegetarian, but a major part of your diet should include these foods.

An article in *Diabetes Care* gives good insight into the importance of vegetables. A study that compared vegetarians with nonvegetarians examined which group developed diabetes more frequently. The study concluded the half of participants who ate the vegetarian diet had nearly 50 percent less diabetes, compared to the participants who ate a nonvegetarian diet.

We can learn several significant factors from this. First is the weight factor. In comparing the BMI of the vegetarians to the BMI of those who ate a typical American diet, the BMI was 23.6 for the vegetarians and 28.8 for the nonvegetarians. That's a five-point spread that tells us a lot about how eating more vegetables is a substantial protection against obesity. Researchers mentioned that other studies confirmed that BMI increases when a wider spectrum of animal products is eaten.

The study also makes an interesting point concerning oxidative stress and chronic inflammation and antioxidants.

Being overweight causes an increase in oxidative stress, which results in chronic inflammation, which in turn causes an increase in insulin resistance. Antioxidants found in vegetables, as well as in fruits, can fight this oxidative stress. This report also found that those who ate the vegetarian diet consumed about one-third more of these protective substances than those who ate the typical American meat diet. Such eating of antioxidants was found to result in a reduction in type 2 diabetes by approximately *40 percent*. Rather than taking a pill, you can just eat your vegetables.

One other significant finding concerning the advantages of eating a lot of vegetables centers on the associated arterial heart disease most diabetics develop. The people who ate mainly vegetables also ate substantially less saturated fat than those who ate the typical American diet. Saturated fat has been shown to increase insulin resistance. Therefore, eating less of the saturated fat so common in meat and dairy products resulted in being more insulin sensitive and less insulin resistant.

I reference this study not to try to get you to become a vegetarian but to emphasize the importance of eating vegetables. It's important to develop this better lifestyle choice now so you can follow it the rest of your life.

High-fiber foods generally let you eat more while consuming fewer calories than those of other foods. If you choose high-fiber foods, you won't have to count calories and you won't have to keep records. You'll base your eating habits on foods that give you the greatest sense of satisfaction as well as having the least number of calories.

The Fat Factor

Remember, there are bad fats and good fats. If you choose a diet based solely on eating protein and eliminating carbohydrates, you open yourself to the associated danger to your arteries from bad fats contained in certain proteins. On some high-protein diets, you can eat all the ham and red meat you want while avoiding most all carbohydrates. Such a diet sounds like a good idea because you're avoiding foods that cause insulin to have to be produced. However, you may be ignoring the risk factors that can cause associated health problems. High-protein foods rich in saturated fat will eventually affect your arteries to the point of risking a heart attack, stroke, Alzheimer's, or even an amputation, as well as putting stress on your kidneys.

An article published in *Diabetes Care* covered an average of 8.8 years and over 37,000 participants who did not have diabetes at the beginning of the study. They found that the ones who ate a higher consumption of total red meat, especially various processed meats such as bacon and hot dogs, had an increased risk of type 2 diabetes.

Why Eat Nuts?

Each gram of fat contains nine calories, and each gram of sugar or protein contains only four. So while you substitute good fat for the bad, you should keep in mind that you're eating more calories when you eat a fat. That aside, several studies point out the advantage of eating nuts if you're diabetic. Nuts are so much better for you than those donuts you used to eat. Just remember to limit the amount because of the calorie content.

The good polyunsaturated and monounsaturated fat in nuts are known to protect against heart attacks in the general population, but what about the diabetic group? Remember that diabetics are at a higher risk of heart attacks than the general population, with more than 80 percent of deaths caused by diseased arteries, resulting in heart attacks or strokes. In contrast, the number of deaths in the general population in America from heart attack or stroke is more than 50 percent. Being diabetic increases those chances significantly.

A study published by the *American Society for Nutrition* compared diabetics who ate at least five servings of nuts per week to those who ate less. Researchers found a significantly lower risk of heart artery disease and heart attacks in the ones who ate more nuts than the ones who ate less. The ones who ate nuts had a higher HDL cholesterol and a lower LDL cholesterol. There was about a 50 percent lower risk of heart attack. Walnuts and almonds are two of the best of the good fat nuts, but peanuts, including peanuts in peanut butter, are the most commonly consumed type of nut in the United States. Peanuts are low in saturated fat and high in monounsaturated and polyunsaturated fat, which have been shown to lower LDL cholesterol and raise HDL cholesterol. Remember, the good fats increase the HDL cholesterol "patrol cars" that drive around and pick up the LDL "splinters" out of the walls of the arteries and carry them to jail, the liver, to be disposed of.

It appears the protective effect of nuts is even greater for diabetics than for nondiabetics. The good fat not only decreases the LDL cholesterol causing plaque in the arteries but also decreases the *inflammation* associated with the disease process going on in the body. This results in a decrease in insulin resistance, which you'll recall is the number one damaging process in the diabetic process.

Researchers concluded that frequent consumption of nuts and peanut butter was associated with a significantly lower heart arterial risk in the individuals who had type 2 diabetes.

A similar report in *Current Diabetes Reports* states that nut consumption was inversely associated with the risk of developing type 2 diabetes. Individuals who consumed one serving of nuts five times per week had a 25 percent lower risk of developing type 2 diabetes compared with the ones who never ate nuts. The study pointed out that one of the protective actions of nuts is reducing insulin resistance.

Why Not Eat Egg Yolk?

For many years, experts told us the dietary cholesterol in egg yolk would cause an increase in our blood cholesterol. Egg yolks were off limits to protect the arteries of your heart. In the past few years, however, that emphasis has been relaxed to some degree, as it became evident that if you're going to concentrate on the culprit of disease of your arteries, you should focus on avoiding saturated fats. Even though the dietary cholesterol may not play as significant a role as once thought, as a diabetic trying to avoid as much saturated fat as possible, you should note that the saturated fat content of egg yolks is higher than you should be eating.

But something about egg yolks in relation to diabetes is not yet completely understood. They have an effect on diabetics different than the effect they have on nondiabetics.

Studies show that if you're diabetic and eat the yolks of eggs, your risk of heart disease significantly increases. This increased risk is substantiated in an article in the *Journal of the American Medical Association*. A study involved thousands of patients who did not have diabetes, artery disease of the heart, or high cholesterol at the beginning of the study. Their egg consumption was broken down to compare the outcome of heart disease in those who ate one egg per day versus those who ate less than one egg per week. The results showed that the ones who ate one egg yolk per day doubled their risk of having heart disease.

It's worth noting that a big part of such an increase in heart risks of diabetics who ate egg yolks is related to the eating habits of people who eat eggs for breakfast. The ones who ate eggs every morning also had the most bacon intake. Also, they were more likely to consume whole milk, red meat, and bread, and less likely to consume skim milk, chicken, vegetables, and fruits.

My mother always told me not to hang around with the wrong crowd. She pointed out three steps to getting into trouble. The first step was just being with boys who may be having a "good" time at a party. "You're in the wrong crowd," she would say. The second step was looking at what they were doing. "Now you're showing interest in the wrong things," she would add. The third step was joining them, becoming part of the wrong party.

The same could be said for eggs. You shouldn't be eating the egg yolk in the first place, but now the crowd that hangs around with the yolk is a problem as well—that bite of bacon or ham, that white-bread toast soaked with butter, and, of course, that cream in your coffee. The best defense is to take my mother's advice. Don't go the egg yolk route to begin with. Eat steel-cut whole grain oatmeal rather than the egg. Add three fruits to the oatmeal and you will be with the right crowd. If you still desire an egg, try a veggie and egg-white omelet. The egg white gives you the taste but doesn't have any saturated fat.

Another article in the *Journal of the American Medical*

Association reports a similar study of the consumption of eggs as related to the risk to the arteries of your heart. It stated that dietary cholesterol found in egg yolk does raise the levels of your LDL cholesterol in your blood, but the effects are relatively small compared to the effects on your arteries caused by the saturated fat found in red meat, cheese, butter, whole milk, and most fried foods. They reported an increased incidence of coronary heart disease, which means disease of the arteries of the heart, among people with diabetes. They pointed out that the consumption of eggs was more detrimental to diabetics than to non-diabetics, and was strongly associated with the mortality of diabetics, especially as related to deaths secondary to heart problems.

One more article that shines a comparable light on whether diabetics should eat eggs was published in *Diabetic Care*. They reviewed several studies, collectively, and concluded that "daily consumption of at least one egg is associated with an increased risk of type 2 diabetes in both men and women, independently of traditional risk factors for type 2 diabetes."

An equally significant part of their report is that daily eating eggs not only increases the risk of diabetes but also increases the risk of heart attacks. The study found a two-fold increased risk of disease of the arteries of the heart in diabetics.

Again, I suggest a high-fiber breakfast such as steel-cut whole grain oatmeal to start your day. You could put a little skim milk on it, of course, plus some high-fiber fruit. And have a cup of coffee rather than the pulp-free orange juice that has no fiber in it.

What about Proteins?

If you're filling up on vegetables and fruits as the largest percentage of your nutrition, what about protein? Most people think meats are the main source of protein in our diet. That's true, but it's a half-truth. Remember that little sign in front of the church that read, "A half-truth is still a whole lie"? Many foods other than animal products have protein, including vegetables, beans, and peas. Weight for weight, a similar amount of protein is in such foods as is found in meat.

In deciding what diet you're going to develop, keep in mind that the cause of death for most diabetics is a heart attack or stroke from disease of the arteries of their heart or brain. Also realize that red meat contains the deadly saturated fat that affects your arteries. Therefore, reduce—or even better, eliminate—red meat protein and replace it with vegetables, beans, and peas for protein.

In summary, focus your new eating habits on getting protein from salads, vegetables, and beans, rather than from meats. Completely avoid red and processed meats, cheese, egg yolks, cream, butter, and fried foods to protect your heart and glucose levels.

Building New Eating Habits

It would be simple if diabetics all had one specific diet plan to follow, but that is not the case. On their website, the American Diabetic Association doesn't give hard-and-fast rules about what foods to eat. Diets like the Mediterranean diet receive favorable reports, but different views on the best diet for diabetics also exist.

Meanwhile, changing habits takes more than dropping a bad habit. You must replace bad habits with good behaviors or you'll return to the bad ones. The best way to change a habit is to choose an alternative, so choose an alternative for each bad food you currently eat.

It helps to record these choices. Write down your menu for each meal of the day. Make your decisions before mealtime. Go over your plans again and again until they become habitual in your mind. Every time you want a snack, know what you're *not* going to let yourself eat even one bite of. If you've been snacking between meals and supplementing it with medication to control the extra sugar you're taking in, get with your doctor and work out a plan where you don't eat the snacks and therefore don't need the extra medication. Plan the amount of food you'll put on your plate in advance, and don't go back for seconds. Decide *before* each lunch and dinner that you will *not* have dessert.

Let me give you a couple of tools to help you in the process of changing your eating habits.

Bad Fats Picture

Visualize a waiter placing a platter with a nice juicy steak in front of you.

Next he places a fried egg, sunny side up, on the steak.

Then he adds a large slice of cheese on top of the egg, and the yolk breaks and runs down over the steak.

To the upper right of the platter is a glass of whole milk, 4 percent of it cream. Such cream represents ice cream, cream-based soups, and the cream sauces restaurants so often place on your food.

To the upper left of your platter is a pat of butter or margarine.

The last part of this mental picture is a small bowl placed at the top of your plate, filled with grease. This last visual represents all fried foods, because most such foods are fried in animal fat.

This whole picture is your saturated fat picture of what causes an influx of the LDL splinters you want to avoid. Begin developing the habit of avoiding such foods like the plague.

Good Fats Picture

Here's a picture to help you remember the good fats. Start with a piece of grilled fish in the center of your plate. Fish such as salmon have the good omega-3 fatty acids. When you think of monounsaturated or polyunsaturated fat, think of fish.

Think of your plate as a clock. At twelve o'clock, you see a small cluster of nuts. It could be almonds or walnuts or peanuts, but just remember that all nuts have good fat.

At the bottom of the clockface, at six o'clock, is an olive. In the Mediterranean diet, a large part of the good fat comes from olive oil. Use olive oil or canola oil when you cook.

At the three o'clock spot are slices of avocado.

In the nine o'clock space are vegetables, high-fiber fruit, beans, or peas.

These are the foods that will help you lose weight and protect your arteries.

Can You Eat Bad Foods in Moderation?

Many articles about diabetes talk about eating certain foods "in moderation." But the only road to successful weight loss and maintaining the loss is abstaining from certain foods, not just eating them in moderation. You must beat the desire for bad foods.

My feeling is that you must beat the desire for dessert, for instance, or you will forever be wanting dessert after each meal and will have to rely on your ability to avoid it. You will have to refight the battle every time you eat lunch and dinner.

To me, the word *moderation* is a trap. It doesn't make sense to "reward" yourself occasionally with the food you're trying to avoid. Most overweight people, diabetic or not, realize the dangers of eating the wrong foods, whether refined sugars in donuts or saturated fat in a nice juicy steak. But what they don't realize is that eating those foods is an addiction. They continue to have a strong desire for that donut or steak and think they can reward themselves occasionally by eating those foods only in moderation. The time eventually comes when they fall back into their addiction and return to eating such foods much more frequently.

The only way to beat an addiction is by abstinence. I remind you, you have to beat the *desire* or you will return to eating the addictive foods you now love to eat. I'm hopeful you'll eliminate the desire for such foods because after reading this book you'll know what each bite is doing to your insulin resistance, blood sugar, and arteries.

General Guidelines for Eating

As mentioned before, even the American Diabetic Association doesn't give a specific diet plan for all diabetics to follow.

Individuals are different and may react differently to a specific diet plan laid out for all diabetics to follow. But you can learn general principles to develop a diet that both covers the glucose problem and protects your arteries.

The *Archives of Internal Medicine* reported on multiple studies that covered almost seventy thousand women who did not have diabetes or heart disease. They were followed for fourteen years to see which type of diet led to becoming diabetic over another type. The diets were divided into two major groups. One group was what they deemed the Western pattern, which included foods such as red meat, processed meat, fried foods, desserts, sweets, French fries, and foods containing refined grains. The other group consisted of the foods you ought to eat—fruits, vegetables, beans, peas, fish, poultry, and whole grains.

You guessed it. The ones who ate the first group of foods had an increased incidence of diabetes of approximately *one and a half times* more than that of the group who ate the foods you're learning to eat in this book.

Another article published in the *Journal of the American College of Nutrition* looks at recommendations from several diabetic organizations worldwide, not just the American Diabetic Association. It takes clinical trials from American, British, and Canadian diabetic associations concerning diets recommended for diabetics and gives us a general overview of the results. No single diet was advised, but in general, most diabetic authorities emphasize:

- A carbohydrate intake of 50 to 60 percent of caloric intake, with higher fiber

- Whole grains, vegetables, fruit, and beans
- An increase in dietary fiber intake
- A restriction of saturated and trans fats

We talked about fiber earlier in this chapter, but note the emphasis on fiber in those results, indicating that a diabetic should consume more fiber than the general population. Again, recall that fiber releases carbohydrates more slowly and allows for easier control of released glucose. If someone recommended a high-carbohydrate diet that included refined sugars found in sweets, drinks, pastries, and desserts, you would never be able to choose that diet.

Remember that whole grains contain the fiber covering of the particular food source. The same is true of many fruits and vegetables that contain integrated fiber. This article specifies that "whole grains, vegetables and fruits are an integral part of the high carbohydrate, high fiber diet."

The key to a carbohydrate diet is the fiber. Write down this list: whole grain breads, cereals, brown rice, beans, peas, nuts, fruits, and vegetables. These foods give you a full feeling with the fewest calories. When you eat this way, you'll see your weight decrease.

Make What You Eat a Habit—and the Right Choice

Breakfast is the easiest meal to make a habit of what you eat. Lunch is almost as easy. If you're eating out, don't look at a menu to choose something new. Look at a menu to find what you're in the habit of eating. The day will come when you won't look at a menu for ten minutes. You'll look at it for one minute, and then out of habit, choose what you've been eating for months or even years. The key is to learn alternatives, and to make your decisions automatic.

But those alternatives must be the right ones. Replace steak with fish. Let a green leafy salad with beans, nuts, and peas and some fish or grilled chicken replace that hamburger for lunch. Choose high-fiber cereal or steel-cut whole-grain oatmeal instead of bacon and eggs and biscuits and gravy. Replace bad with good. Create new eating habits so you won't have to "decide" whether you want steak or fish. You won't have to think about whether to eat the cheese, or the buttered toast, or the high-fat salad dressing.

Your new habits will change what you want to eat. I assure you, it will be surprising how your desire for certain foods changes. You may find it hard to believe now, but the day will come when someone brags on how good a cinnamon roll is, but you won't have a moment of desire to taste the icing. The habits you begin developing now will make it easier and easier to defeat those moments of temptation.

Rules of Thumb

Again, you will read conflicting information about high-carbohydrate/low-fat diets as well as low-carb/high-fat diets. Whichever diet you follow, the important point is to control your sugar and protect the arteries of your heart.

Below are some dietary "rules of thumb" Dr. Ross Tanner, a physician in Alaska who treats diabetics, has developed to help his patients not only control their sugar but also protect their arteries. It's good reading for them, and I think it will be for you also.

The three basic nutrient groups are carbohydrate, fat, and protein. Each group has health advantages and disadvantages. If you're diabetic, carbohydrates can raise your blood sugar. Whether or not you're diabetic, eating too much carbohydrate and fat will make you gain weight. Eating too much carbohydrate and fat can also make your blood cholesterol numbers worse, which is bad for your heart. As you know, there are good fats and bad fats, good carbohydrates and bad carbohydrates. The good fats are in fish, nuts, and olive oil, while the bad fats include the trans fats found in red meat, cheese, cream, butter, and fried foods. The good fats are heart healthy while the bad fats play havoc on the arteries throughout your body.

Remember, ounce per ounce, beans have as much protein as red meat. The good carbohydrates are in the foods with high fiber, while the bad carbs are found in refined sugar foods.

Try to follow the guidelines below when planning your menus.

1. Bad carbohydrates (watch the portion sizes of all carbohydrates)
   Avoid white starches: sugar, bread and other flour products, rice, potatoes, pasta, noodles
   Avoid root vegetables: potatoes, sweet potatoes, yams, parsnips, turnips, and beets
   Avoid high-sugar, low-fiber fruits: watermelon, honeydew melon, cantaloupe, grapes, pineapple, raisins, dates, mango, papaya, kiwi, commercial fruit cocktail, and fruit juices
   Avoid sweet corn, pumpkin, and squash

Avoid does not mean abstain; it means better choices exist with regard to consuming certain carbohydrates based on glycemic index and fiber content.

2. Good carbohydrates

Good vegetable choices: baked beans, other legumes (butter beans, chickpeas, kidney beans, lima beans, lentils, pinto beans, peas, and others), broccoli, cauliflower, string beans, spinach, cabbage, brussels sprouts, kale, peppers, radishes, celery, and other green vegetables

Good fruit choices: apples, pears, apricots, peaches, plums, cherries, grapefruit, oranges, strawberries, blueberries, blackberries, and raspberries

3. Good fats

Good fat choices: salmon, olive oil, canola oil, safflower oil, sunflower oil, olives, nuts, peanuts, and avocados

4. Proteins

Good protein choices: beans and other legumes, egg whites, soy and tofu products, fish, white meat poultry

Sample Daily Menus

Breakfast

Steel-cut oatmeal with whole-grain toast

Raspberries

Bananas

Blueberries

High-fiber whole-grain cereal with skim milk

Peaches

Strawberries

Raspberries

Lunch

Green leafy salad with fat-free dressing

Beans

Nuts

Peas

Pears

Apples

Add salmon or grilled chicken

Dinner

Salad

Salmon or grilled chicken

Vegetable plate from high-fiber table below

High-Fiber Foods

Almonds 18 grams per cup	Apples 4.4 grams
Asparagus 4 grams per cup	Avocados 13.6 grams
Bananas 3.1 grams	Black beans 15 grams per cup
Blackberries 7.6 grams per cup	Broccoli 5.1 grams per cup
Brussels sprouts 4.1 grams per cup	Carrots 3.6 grams per cup
Collard greens 8 grams per cup	Green beans 4 grams per cup

Green peas 14.4 grams per cup

Kidney beans 11.4 grams per cup

Lima beans 13.2 grams per cup

Pears 5.5 grams

Raspberries 8 grams per cup

Steel-cut oats 20 grams per cup

Kale 3 grams per cup

Lettuce 1 gram per cup

Navy beans 19.2 grams per cup

Peas 8.8 grams per cup

Spinach 4 grams per cup

Whole-grain bread 4–5 grams per slice

11. The Importance of Ideal Weight

I'm asked these questions numerous times: "How do I figure my ideal weight? How do I measure it?"

We've used two terms in this book: BMI (body mass index) and ideal weight. BMI is a good number to look at for overall purposes, especially if you're doing a medical study. But if you're looking at your individual specific goal weight, a better target is to determine your ideal weight. Let's look at the difference between BMI and ideal weight.

The National Institutes of Health uses BMI as the defining line of whether your weight is in a normal, overweight, or obese range. It's calculated using your height and weight. Medical studies use BMI to compare people who are of normal weight or above normal weight. The normal category is below 25 BMI, overweight is 25 to 30, and obese is over 30. The problem is these ranges don't identify an ideal weight for a particular person because of a twenty- to thirty-pound variance. You can be twenty to thirty pounds above your ideal weight and still fall within the "normal" range, but being at a normal BMI doesn't necessarily mean you're at your ideal weight.

Two-thirds of Americans fall within the overweight or obese category, but only 12 percent are at their ideal weight. Your goal should be to reach your ideal weight.

How to Figure Ideal Weight

First, be more precise than the BMI scale. Everyone is different. Some are heavy boned or heavily built. Some are much more muscular than others, and muscle mass weighs more than fat tissue. Some are petite. No absolute way to state your ideal weight in exactly x number of pounds exists, but there is a scale more exact than BMI.

The formula I like best is one that fine-tunes the BMI scale. It's based on your height and weight, and I call it the *ideal body mass index*. It gives you a much better idea of where to aim.

Men use 105 pounds as the base weight number for five feet. For every inch over five feet, add five pounds. Ideal weight for a five-foot-seven-inch male would be 140 pounds.

Women use 95 pounds as the base weight number for five feet. For every inch over five feet, add four pounds. Ideal weight for a five-foot-seven-inch female would be 123 pounds.

Using the ideal weight scale, you must consider personal body build differences you may have and add pounds accordingly. This is especially true with men. So adding five to fifteen pounds to your ideal weight number may be appropriate. My best advice when you get near that ideal weight number is to stand in front of a full-length mirror and turn sideways to see if you have a lower abdominal pouch sticking out. The image in the mirror tells it all. (That's what I tell my overweight friends who tell me they're at "normal" weight, and there's a lot of truth to it.)

As you begin to move toward your ideal weight, you can be encouraged by the effect of weight reduction on the health of your heart arteries and the disease of the heart in individuals with type 2 diabetes. The *Look AHEAD Trial,* presented in *Diabetes Care,* consisted of 5,145 individuals with type 2 diabetes with a BMI over 25. In other words, they were all either overweight or obese. Their goal was to lose 7 percent of their initial body weight. The study was first reported one year after the trial began, and then again after four years of follow-up. One group had individual meetings to achieve and maintain weight loss through a decrease in the number of calories eaten as well as increased physical activity. Their main exercise was walking.

The second group had only support and educational meetings, information concerning diabetes, and did not do the physical activity.

The exercise group lost an average of 8.6 percent of their initial weight, while the non-exercise group lost only 0.7 percent. That factor alone speaks loudly about the importance of including exercise in your decision to lose extra weight.

While those stats affirm the importance of weight loss, the focus of this study was on health issues of the heart, which are related to diabetes. The group that lost weight through diet and exercise not only had improvement in blood sugar, but also had a reduction in high blood pressure, better cholesterol numbers, and improved kidney function numbers.

The medications for their diabetes, blood pressure, and cholesterol were all reduced. Overall, researchers concluded there was a 21 percent improvement in the condition of the heart and arteries in the group that exercised. The authors concluded, "The modest increase in physical activity, primarily walking, had a very beneficial effect on weight loss and diabetic control."

That shows the choices you make can significantly influence the heart and artery risk factors associated with diabetes. The study also showed that any weight loss led to improvements. The report supplied substantial evidence that even modest weight losses of 5 to 10 percent of initial weight produce significant, clinically relevant improvements in the associated heart risks. Even those who lost just 2 to 5 percent of their weight had significant improvement in their risk factor numbers. Those who lost 5 to 10 percent had even greater odds of improvement than those who lost the 2 to 5 percent, and those who lost 10 to 15 percent had even greater odds of improvement than the group that lost 5 to 10 percent.

The greater the weight change, the greater the improvement of their glucose control, drop in blood pressure, and increase in their HDL cholesterol.

Are You Committed?

Now comes the real question that will determine whether you do all you can to physically develop a different you, from a weight standpoint.

Are you committed? No one else can make that determination for you, no matter how much they would like to see you succeed. Commitment doesn't come in stages; you're either in or out. You either will or you won't. It's pretty black and white.

I tell you, if you wholeheartedly commit, you'll indeed reach your ideal weight. There is a tremendous difference between *deciding* to lose weight and *committing* to lose weight.

I was sitting in church one Sunday when the pastor asked everyone who had ever decided to go on a diet to lose weight to raise their hand. I couldn't believe how many hands went up. Maybe all but about 5 percent of the congregation admitted to dieting (and I bet those 5 percent didn't tell the truth about other things either). There was some laughter as so many people who were overweight raised their hands, probably because their *decision* hadn't produced results. It wasn't the same as *commitment*.

If you commit to something, you must concentrate on some big things as well as on some small things to be successful.

I weigh myself every morning, and I'm surprised at the variance from one day to the next. My eating is mostly consistent, I exercise six days a week, and I have been within one to two pounds of my goal weight for years. I have a few rules I follow to keep my weight consistent. If I'm a half pound above my ideal weight, I go back to my "weight loss" eating habits. I don't eat anything between meals or after dinner. My meals will typically be salads for both lunch and dinner, with some fish or grilled chicken on the salad. Of course, I consume no calories from beverages.

I admit that I may get a twinge of hunger sometime during the afternoon, so I apply "the ten-minute factor." I fill my stomach with a noncaloric drink and begin doing something else with my time. I may send a text or email or call someone, but the point is I get busy doing something that gets my mind on anything besides wanting to snack.

I have practiced this plan for years to control my weight day by day. I didn't want to weigh only once a week and then realize I was three pounds overweight and had to go back to my weight-loss lifestyle for many days to catch up.

I developed this plan on my own, and I had not seen anything similar until I read an article by the National Weight Control Registry. Researchers selected a group of over three thousand members who had lost over thirty pounds and had kept it off for over a year. This successful weight-loss group typically reported that they ate a low-fat/low-calorie diet. Four-fifths of them ate breakfast every day. They exercised and reported watching less television than the norm. They reported that those who weighed themselves daily had a decreased risk of weight regain. The main reason for this is that frequent weighing provides an opportunity for positive reinforcement of weight control for that day.

These individuals were placed into one of three groups. Thirty-six percent of the group weighed themselves daily, 42 percent at least weekly, and 21 percent less than once a week. The bottom line of the study was that "those individuals who weighed themselves daily were 82% more likely to maintain their weight loss compared with those who weighed less often." In addition to that, they found that starting to weigh themselves less frequently was associated with greater weight regain.

Those who weighed daily were able to identify small weight gains and *immediately* make appropriate changes. For those whose weight was maintained, daily weighing was a positive reinforcement.

The Secret to Maintaining Your Weight Loss

You've heard that the most crucial factor in defeating diabetes is weight loss. But that's not the whole truth. The most crucial factor in defeating diabetes is *maintaining* the weight loss. I have many overweight friends and acquaintances who are working on losing the excess. It's so exciting to see someone after several months who's lost a significant amount of weight. On the other hand, it's close to depressing to see anyone regain their weight.

Almost any weight-loss plan "works," usually temporarily. The challenge is keeping the weight off. One of the saddest statistics in medical literature is that only 2 to 20 percent of people who lose weight maintain that weight loss. Weight loss is your first step, but the key step for optimal health is maintaining your ideal weight.

Here is the secret to the eating plan in this book: develop eating habits as you lose the weight that you can continue for the rest of your life. Remember, food is an addiction. The bad foods that play havoc with diabetes are foods you have become addicted to, like desserts.

One diabetic told me she ate only one bite of her husband's chocolate cake at a party they attended. "One bite. That satisfied me." I didn't want to go into sermon mode, so I didn't explain that she didn't realize she was addicted to chocolate. I'm not a betting man, but if I were, I would have bet anyone in the room that she would be eating a whole piece of chocolate cake sometime down the line. My favorite analogy is that saying one bite of a "bad" food you're addicted to is like someone who smokes saying one puff of a cigarette will satisfy them for a week. Addiction doesn't work that way. Abstinence is essential to beating addiction. As I've mentioned before, if you abstain for sixty days, the desire for that particular food will be greatly diminished to the point that you can control it. Remember that number— *sixty* days of abstinence to beat the food addiction.

Let's look at some more information from the National Weight Control Registry. To join the program, you must have lost at least thirty pounds and kept it off for at least a year. The average participant has lost sixty-six pounds and kept it off for five and a half years. Ninety-eight percent of the participants report that they changed their dieting lifestyle in some way to lose weight. Ninety-four percent increased their physical activity, and the most frequent form of exercise was walking. Diet and exercise were the keys to success.

Most of them state they've kept weight off by maintaining a low-calorie/low-fat diet and with high levels of activity. Ninety percent of the participants exercise, on average, about one hour per day. Seventy-eight percent eat breakfast every day, and seventy-five percent weigh themselves at least once a week.

More than ten thousand members are enrolled in the study, and they complete annual questionnaires about their weight, diet, and exercise. Their responses give us a good example of how a large group of individuals were able to keep their weight off. I like to study success and find out how it's been accomplished. I think we can get a lot of good advice on losing weight and sustaining that loss in diabetics. Ninety-eight percent of the people reduced their intake of food. Some of this would be by reducing the size of portions, some by cutting out snacks, and some by eliminating desserts, which are all excess calories.

One number I especially like is that 94 percent of them increased their exercise. That says so much. Only 10 percent of them reported losing their weight by diet alone. Exercise is so important. That's why it's step one in our plan.

Since weight is such a factor in causing and preventing diabetes, I like to dig into what has been successful with weight loss and apply it to diabetes. Let's look at a report the National Weight Control Registry published in an article in the *American Journal of Clinical Nutrition.* This study focused on long-term weight-loss maintenance. The weight is lost. It's not found again.

Here are some practices that made them succeed. They engaged in high levels of physical activity for approximately an hour a day. The majority ate a low-fat/low-calorie diet and ate breakfast every day. That diet is similar to what you've read about in this book, including fiber found in fruits and vegetables, beans, and whole grains, while avoiding the saturated fat in red meats, cheese, butter, cream, and fried foods.

Participants also weighed themselves frequently.

Finally, they were consistent in their dieting. They ate the same way on weekends and holidays as they did the rest of the week. In other words, they developed eating habits they could continue day after day and year after year. They didn't "reward" themselves on weekends or holidays with "bads." They developed a good diet and made that their habit. The ones who stuck to their habits, including weekends and holidays, were one and a half times more likely to maintain their weight over the subsequent year than participants who allowed themselves to change their diet on weekends and holidays. The authors of the study summed up the findings by stating that "individuals who allowed themselves more flexibility on holidays had greater risk of weight regain."

Allowing flexibility in your eating lifestyle creates more opportunities for loss of control. If you don't develop eating habits that you'll follow consistently, you'll slip back into old eating styles. This study confirms that. Very few of the participants who neglected their eating habits and regained even small amounts of weight were able to recover from the slip. The study also stated, "Individuals who maintain a consistent diet regimen across the week and year appear more likely to maintain their weight loss over time."

There's More to Excess Fat Than Looks

Because you've been reading this book, you already know most of the bottom lines the following studies reveal. But every study should make you more and more determined to commit to fighting your diabetes with lifestyle changes. They should help you get past the idea that losing weight is mostly about looks, if that's what you've been thinking for years.

An article in the *New England Journal of Medicine* said it best: "Excess body fat is the single most important determinant of type 2 diabetes." Many diabetic patients are told they should reduce their weight, but that's about as far as it goes. Doctors know the significance of excess body fat in the role of diabetes. The physician feels obligated to explain this to their patient, but then the need to treat diabetes immediately comes into play. Rather than beginning the patient on exercise, a healthy eating program, and weight loss, the doctor usually starts with medication to control the patient's blood glucose immediately. This can create a false sense of security, and the patient begins relying on whatever medication the doctor prescribes.

There's another way. Yes, your doctor must go to work on controlling your glucose, but I'm emphasizing that you must go to work changing your lifestyle habits to beat the disease.

Excess weight is one of the major factors in developing insulin resistance. Adipose tissue produces and secretes certain chemicals that cause an inflammatory response at the cell surfaces that prevents insulin from being able to function properly. Without going too deep into the medical process, a protein is found in the blood whenever an inflammatory response is going on in the body, which can measure this inflammation. This protein is called the C-reactive Protein. This is one of the proteins elevated in overweight patients who are prediabetic or diabetic. With more inflammation is a greater amount of C-reactive Protein, showing the relationship of excess weight and inflammation, resulting in insulin resistance.

Being overweight and developing diabetes are connected. The journal article mentioned above points out that obesity and weight gain, along with being physically inactive, dramatically increase the risk of diabetes. The study included over eighty-four thousand women who did not have diabetes or heart disease at the beginning of the study and followed them to see which ones were more prone to developing diabetes.

The researchers set up a guideline for diet as well as exercise. They pointed to earlier studies that showed a reduced risk of type 2 diabetes in people who had a higher intake of cereal fiber and polyunsaturated fat and an increase in diabetes in those who ate saturated fat and a high-glycemic load. This report emphasized eating high-fiber carbohydrates, where the glucose is released slowly or not at all, as well as eating good polyunsaturated fat found in fish, nuts, and olives rather than the bad fat found in red meat, butter, cream, and fried foods. The participants who ate more of the bad foods and were overweight had higher C-reactive Protein in their blood, which pointed to higher amounts of inflammation.

This study took an even stricter range on body mass index. Most studies use a BMI below 25 as delineating the normal range, 25 to 30 as being overweight, and above 30 as being obese. The results of this study showed that a BMI at the high end of the normal range of 23.0 to 24.9 was associated with a substantially higher risk of diabetes than a BMI less than 23.0. Being overweight increases inflammation.

The journal *Diabetes Care* put it succinctly: "If you are overweight, your odds for developing diabetes are two-fold greater than a normal BMI and if your BMI is in the obese range, you will have a four-fold greater chance of developing diabetes."

The study reported in the *New England Journal of Medicine*, which used stricter BMI than the usual, is just a reminder that if you use BMI as your gauge, there can be a twenty- to thirty-pound variance with your particular height and body build. A report in the *Canadian Journal of Diabetes* pointed this out concerning the significance of weight as related to BMI. They did a collective review of medical reports covering over 900,000 adults and concluded that for each five points body mass index above 25, there was an associated approximately 30 percent higher overall mortality. The more overweight you are, the more chance you'll come to the end of life before you should.

Their findings showed it wasn't just BMI overweight that increased your chances of diabetes and early mortality; a lack of exercise also was associated with a significantly increased risk of diabetes even when excluding BMI.

The next sentence may be the most important sentence in this book: *The main factor they highlighted in their concluding remarks suggested that 87 percent of the new cases of diabetes that developed during the study might have been prevented if all the women had done what the women in the low-risk group had done.* That should get your attention and encourage you to develop the same lifestyles of eating and exercising to lose weight as the low-risk group did.

One of the focuses of the study was to see how many of the individuals could have prevented becoming diabetic by weighing less. Remembering that an *overweight* BMI is from 25 to 30, approximately half of the individuals in this category could have avoided diabetes. In evaluating those who were in the *obese* category of a BMI of 30 and above, they could have reduced their risk of developing diabetes by 24 percent if they had followed the eating and exercising guidelines in the control group.

Their overall conclusion was astonishing. They stated that weight control was the most effective way to reduce the risk of type 2 diabetes. Another important conclusion says these same guidelines of proper eating, weight loss, and exercise were associated with an 83 percent reduction in the associated heart disease found in diabetics.

To emphasize this correlation of excess weight and diabetes, consider this review from *The Obesity Society* publication. The opening sentence caught my eye: "The single best predictor of type 2 diabetes is overweight or obesity." The medical community doesn't fully understand the cause and workings of diabetes. For instance, most diabetics are overweight or obese, but some people who aren't obese have diabetes. So when we look at the numbers of how weight affects you if you're diabetic, remember to focus more on how you personally fit into those statistics. In other words, if you're overweight, look at what studies say about the connection between being overweight and becoming diabetic or having diabetes. This report puts it succinctly: "Almost ninety percent of people living with type 2 diabetes are overweight or have obesity."

This report studied individuals who were overweight, and the researchers state being overweight causes an added pressure on the body's ability to use insulin to properly control blood sugar levels, and those who are overweight are therefore more likely to develop diabetes.

Whether you have diabetes or prediabetes, this report should encourage you to get to an ideal weight, especially because the study concludes, "Type 2 diabetes is largely preventable."

This article pointed out that many other studies have shown repeatedly that even a modest amount of weight loss in the 5 to 10 percent range can delay or even prevent the development of type 2 diabetes among those who have associated risks that go along with diabetes. Even moderate weight loss plus moderate exercise, such as walking for thirty minutes a day, five days a week, reduced the development of diabetes by 40 to 60 percent in studies that lasted three to six years.

This statement summarizes the above article well: "Weight management is the best thing you can do to prevent the development of diabetes."

Whether prediabetic or diabetic, managing your weight must be foremost in your mind, along with the knowledge that exercise is the one best lifestyles you can develop. Exercise will not only allow you to accomplish that weight loss, but allow you to sustain your ideal weight for years to come.

Are you convinced yet? It's not just about looks. It's about your health. You can do many things to improve your life if you're prediabetic or diabetic. Remember, we're not simply talking about extra years to live; we're talking about extra *active* years to enjoy life to the fullest. You don't want to go through the rest of your life fighting the complications associated with having diabetes. Commit to change your lifestyle today so you can have those enjoyable future years.

Six Secrets to Losing Weight

You're committed to getting to an ideal weight. How do you do it? So many weight-loss books and advertisements show people losing weight, telling us the "real secret" to losing and keeping it off. I will admit that such weight-loss schemes can work. You will lose weight with any of them, but only 2 percent of the people who lose it are able to maintain the loss. If you want to maintain your good work, develop the kind of eating lifestyle in losing your weight that allows you to continue those same eating habits after you've reached your ideal weight. You stay on the same basic diet out of habit from then on.

To lose weight, your body must expend more energy than it takes in. You may be relieved to know that, with the approach you're learning in this book, you don't have to count calories, but you do have to learn which foods have the fewest calories and which ones contain the most. You'll also need to know how many calories you burn as you exercise.

Carbohydrates and proteins contain four calories per gram, while fats contain nine. That's why diets high in fat can lead to a greater weight gain. That's why a plate full of carbohydrates and protein will lead to less weight gain than one full of fatty foods. We will get into more detail, but that's a good start for our discussion.

Earlier I told you the secret to fighting your diabetes with how you manage food is to develop an eating plan you can follow not only as you lose weight, but for the rest of your life. Now let's look at some specific secrets for losing weight. In them, you'll see some of the same factors and advice in the book thus far, but in six simple steps.

Secret #1: Skip Snacks

Snacks are extra calories. In the weight-loss phase of your plan, they're completely excluded. Learn what to eat at meals so you won't crave a snack between them. If you're on medication, discuss with your doctor how to regulate that specific medication when you develop a habit of eating three meals a day and no snacks in between. Your doctor may lower the dose so you won't have to eat between meals because your insulin dose was more than needed.

Why is a snack so detrimental to weight loss? Without going into detail about what takes place in your body, here's a quick explanation.

Let's say three hours or so after eating a meal your blood sugar drops below its normal level because your insulin has allowed your body to use some of the glucose. Your body is going to get the needed glucose one way or another. It will either begin throwing switches that break down fat-energy and other substances in your body to convert them to glucose, or you will eat a snack your body quickly absorbs and converts to glucose. Your body will begin burning calories from the snack rather than breaking the stored energy down into the needed glucose. You don't have to be a physician to understand you're going to burn more calories from your body if you don't eat the snack.

Later in this chapter we'll talk about snacks and "fake hunger."

Secret #2: Employ the Ten-Minute Factor

How do you avoid snacks? The secret is the ten-minute factor. I told you earlier that this is one way I control my own weight, and this is how you can train yourself in self-control too. Willpower is a learnable skill. Each victory adds up to new eating habits.

Again, food is an addiction. It must be addressed the same way you would control any other addiction. To beat an addiction, you must beat the desire. You can't decide to stop eating snacks by just wanting to stop. You can't control the desire to eat a particular snack at a particular time simply with self-control. But you can control that desire for about ten minutes.

159

Here's the ten-minute secret to avoiding snacks:

Step one: tell yourself you're not going to eat that particular snack you want for the next ten minutes.

Step two: drink a glass of noncaloric liquid: a glass of iced tea, a cup of coffee, water—anything that has zero calories. Get some liquid into your stomach.

Step three: do something else. Make a phone call or read something. Take your cup of coffee to a colleague's desk and talk about your work or any other item of interest. Go outside for a short walk. Do anything other than taking a bite of that snack.

You'll beat that desire for that snack for at least ten minutes and then be able to resist completely. The first few times you employ the ten-minute factor, it may be a little difficult, but it is doable. After you do it several times, it will become easier and easier to break that snack habit. Before long, you will be practicing the ten-minute factor out of habit. Each time you do it, you'll be developing small actions that will change your habits related to snacks. The accumulation of ten-minute factor victories will give you a sense of success.

Secret #3: Forgo Desserts

Desserts are first cousins to snacks. In the weight-loss phase, your decision about dessert must be to never have any. Again, you have an addiction, and to beat an addiction, you must beat the desire. As I've said, it takes sixty days of abstinence to break the desire pattern of your mind. After that time, it doesn't mean you never desire the particular food you've not eaten for sixty days, but it does mean that after sixty days you'll be able to control that desire. Before too much longer, that desire for dessert will grow weaker and weaker. I assure you, the day will come when you're eating out with friends when dessert time comes, and you'll order a cup of coffee or tea and just enjoy the company while they eat dessert.

You can't beat the desire for desserts with moderation. Eating only one or two bites of chocolate cake won't work. To lose weight, avoid every extra calorie you can, and avoid desserts like the plague.

Secret #4: Choose the Right Foods

As I've mentioned before, carbohydrates and protein contain four calories per gram and fats contain nine calories per gram. Knowing that formula makes it easier to avoid fats. The heart of our weight-loss plan is learning which foods fill you up with the least number of calories. These are the foods you want to get into the habit of eating. A simple rule of thumb is to choose vegetables as your primary food, with beans and peas secondary, and then adding high-fiber fruit. Beans have as much protein per weight as beef. Salads will become a mainstay for your meals, with the addition of fish or chicken. A vegetable plate for lunch or dinner is perfect.

Vegetables, high-fiber fruit, whole grains, beans, and peas give you that full feeling. You can fill up on them and yet be ingesting fewer calories, which allows you to lose weight.

At the same time, avoid the bad fats that come with red meat, cheese, butter, cream, and fried foods, not to mention avoiding fatty salad dressings and the creamy sauces they pour over food in restaurants.

Again, I remind you to talk to your physician as you develop your new eating lifestyle to ensure your glucose levels stay in proper proportion. You'll be checking your blood glucose between meals. With your physician's help, rather than having too much medication on board and having to take some sugar to get your glucose level back up, you will be taking less and less medication and not eating between meals.

This is a good time to train yourself to remove the wrong foods from your kitchen and anywhere else you might have them. Don't have the wrong food within sight or reach. The best example I know came from a gentleman who made the commitment to begin eating the right foods and not eating the bad. I had explained the foods that harmed his arteries—the red meat, cheese, cream, butter, and fried foods. He seemed serious about changing his eating habits, but I knew he was earnest when I saw him the next day.

We were passing in the hallway when he stopped me and said, "Last night I got to thinking about what you explained concerning the danger of saturated fat." He looked me square in my eyes and continued with a half-smile, half-smirk. "I just want you to know what I did. I took a gallon container of ice cream out of my freezer and threw it in the trash. It was my favorite ice cream; 28 percent butterfat type. But I threw it away." He laughed and started walking away, but then he looked back at me. "Just wanted you to know."

I encourage you to do likewise.

Once you get your cupboards, refrigerator, and freezer free of bad foods, the best way to keep them that way is to be specific when grocery shopping. You'll be surprised at the difference you can make by making the right decisions when you shop, especially if you have a list you stick to. Choose the foods that don't harm your arteries. Avoid those saturated fats.

As you develop your new eating habits, you will also realize the role fiber plays in controlling your blood sugar. Remember that high-fiber carbohydrates keep the sugar contained. The fiber is like a woven cage that lets the glucose out a little at a time. That's why eating whole-grain steel-cut oatmeal for breakfast will keep you from getting hungry before lunchtime. The fiber in the full-kernel oats gives you a full feeling and lets the carbohydrates break down slowly throughout the morning. Similar is the difference between whole-grain breads and white breads. They both release sugar, but the whole-grain has the fiber that will release the sugar more slowly and not give that spike in your blood sugar level. The slow release is similar with the vegetable plate you eat for lunch or the large salad with beans, peas, nuts, or vegetables you eat at dinner.

In the weight-loss part of your new lifestyle, think of bread as extra sugar. Once into your weight-maintaining diet, you'll begin eating whole-grain foods, including bread, but in your weight-loss phase, cut out all breads. I saw a diabetic order a sandwich and French fries for lunch. The bun on the sandwich was huge. It was so thick that they stuck a knife through, from top to bottom. It stood straight up with the handle sticking out the top of the sandwich. I'm sure he was taking the proper amount of medication to cover such a lunch. But even after you get to your goal weight, you shouldn't eat foods similar to eating sugar, and white bread and potatoes are two such foods.

If you're going to eat dry toast with your steel-cut oatmeal after you get to your ideal weight, eat whole-grain toast.

The bottom line is that rather than counting calories, learn the proper foods. Write down each basic meal for the day and build your eating habits around a core of healthy meal options.

Secret #5: Eat Nothing Fried

Frying a food adds about a third more calories. You get not only extra calories from the fat in the oil, but the oil will most likely be animal fat, which will cause your LDL cholesterol to increase. If you're going to use a cooking oil at home, use olive oil or canola oil, which are good fats despite giving you extra calories.

Secret #6: Exercise

You get more benefit from exercise in losing weight than simply burning a certain number of calories. A rule of thumb is that you burn one hundred calories per mile, whether you walk or jog. Of course, it will take longer to burn a hundred calories if you're walking, but walking is a hundredfold better than not exercising at all. Once again, remember the study performed at Brown University, which divided a group of women into two groups. Both groups were placed on the same weight-loss diet. One group exercised, and the other didn't. The outcome said a lot: *the group that exercised lost almost twice the weight as the group that only dieted.*

It's true that exercise burns calories, but it also does more. Exercise takes a lot of commitment, even more than it takes to not eat a certain food.

Exercise is the ultimate commitment you make to yourself when you decide to lose weight. If you commit to exercising five to six days a week, it will affect all the other factors that result in weight loss. As I've said before, exercise tells your mind that you're serious about the new lifestyle you're undertaking. Exercise reinforces all the other weight-loss factors. So whether you decide to walk, run, swim, ride a bicycle, or begin strength training, you're on the right path to success. I'll say it again: exercise is so important that I place it as step number one in beginning your victory over diabetes.

These six simple secrets are all attainable, and you will see weight-loss success as you replace your old habits with new ones based on these secrets. Before long, you'll be eating a routine breakfast of steel-cut oatmeal or a high-fiber cereal with some fruit. If you eat lunch out, it will take only a minute to find a vegetable plate or a salad with grilled chicken or salmon. Your dinner will become fairly predictable. It may not sound all that exciting, but once you beat the desire for bad foods and begin eating good foods, your food addictions will be of the past, your tastes will change, and you will enjoy your new, healthier lifestyle.

I've mentioned them before, but let me throw in two sneaky little enemies to be on the lookout for as you develop your new eating habits. They both not only affect your weight, but your heart.

One is cheese—that beloved food I told you I eliminated from my own diet. If you eat at home, it's easy to completely do away with eating cheese. But if you eat out, remember that cheese is added to a lot of what you order unless you specify "no cheese"—especially to salads. Unless you tell your waiter no cheese, you will invariably find they have sprinkled cheese on top.

I even had it happen to me when I ordered a veggie egg-white omelet. I thought I had covered all my bases when I told them I wanted dry whole-wheat toast—no butter. But I was surprised when I took the first bite of my omelet. They had placed cheese in the middle of it, which had obviously melted throughout all the vegetables. I don't like to send back food at a restaurant, but that was one time I had to ask them to remake my order with no cheese.

Another item to be aware of as you lose that excess weight is salad dressing. Not only do salad dressings add extra calories, but so many of them are loaded with saturated fat. Make sure you're using either a nonfat dressing or an olive oil or vinaigrette type. And be sure salads in restaurants don't come to you with dressing already on them.

Once you get to your ideal weight, you can make some changes to your eating plans. Your portions may become a little larger, or you may want to have a snack, choosing a high-fiber fruit or some nuts. Those changes will come in the future, but right now, do all you can to beat the desire for wrong foods.

Does Skipping Breakfast Help You Lose Weight?

Skipping breakfast is an increasing trend in America, where over 25 percent of people do it. Some people skip breakfast because they believe they're reducing their overall calorie intake and by so doing are helping their weight loss. But an article in the journal *Obesity Research* points out this may or may not be the case.

Researchers examined short-term studies on the role of breakfast and energy balance and found mixed results. Some of the studies showed lower total intake of calories in non-breakfast eaters while other studies supported that those who skip breakfast tend to eat more calorie-dense foods later in the day. In other words, if you skip breakfast, you tend to eat a heavier lunch because you're hungrier.

As pointed out in this particular study, the National Weight Control Registry group of successful weight-loss maintainers ate breakfast most mornings. Seventy-eight percent ate breakfast every morning, but almost 95 percent ate breakfast most days of the week. Fewer than 5 percent never ate breakfast.

These statistics make me want to eat breakfast every morning.

The "Fake Hunger Syndrome"

Most people who lose weight eat three meals a day: breakfast, lunch, and dinner, and again, I recommend avoiding snacks completely when you're working on weight loss. That's why it's so important to eat high-fiber foods where the glucose is released slowly over a longer period rather than a quick release and a spike in blood sugar resulting in a spike in insulin needed, followed by too large a drop in blood glucose, which may signal to you that you need a snack. And again, it's important to check with your doctor about medication control as you develop your new eating habits.

Let's look at what takes place in your body when you eat a meal. This will help you understand what happens when you have a slight hunger sensation a few hours after you eat and want to eat a snack to satisfy that hunger. That hunger feeling may be fake hunger.

Step 1. Soon after your first bite of food, some carbohydrates are digested and broken down into sugar. This increase of glucose in your blood signals the pancreas to begin producing insulin. The insulin is like the key that unlocks the door of your cells to open, allowing the glucose particles to enter the cell to be used as energy.

Step 2. Any excess sugar in the blood is stored in the liver or muscles as glycogen.

Step 3. As time passes, the glucose in your bloodstream is fully used and no more digestible glucose is available. At this point, you may begin to have a little sense of hunger because the sugar in the blood has been used up and your blood sugar level is lower. When this happens, the body turns the switch on in the liver to begin releasing and breaking down the stored glycogen back into glucose, which goes back into the bloodstream to furnish nutrition to the cells of the body. This process is called glycolysis, meaning the stored glycogen is beginning to break back down into glucose. At that point, our bodies feed off the stored glycogen rather than glucose from additional food.

Step 4. When the stored glycogen begins to be completely used up, the body must get glucose from somewhere. Now, many hours after your meal, true hunger comes into play. The glucose from food recently eaten has all been used, the glucose from the stored glycogen has been used, and a warning bell rings, telling you to eat some food to restart the cycle at step 1. If you checked your glucose level, you would find you were at a true low level of glucose. If you don't eat now, a process called gluconeogenesis begins because the glycogen stores have been depleted.

Where does fake hunger fit into your body's need for glucose? It's important to understand how and when this happens so you don't let a feeling of hunger make you think you need something to eat between meals. When you first begin changing your habits, you may have to check your blood sugar to make certain you're still in the normal glucose range and that you haven't given yourself too much insulin or other medication that dropped your glucose too low. Once you get that worked out, you'll be able to balance your medications to fit a plan that will let you skip those extra calories in snacks, which prevent you from losing weight.

When you experience fake hunger in step 3, this is not the time to eat snacks. Additional glucose will come either from eating a snack, from the glycogen breakdown, or through gluconeogenesis. Let your body work properly so that the needed energy comes from what you have already eaten rather than adding new food and additional calories to the equation.

I like to simplify the above example by looking at that fall in blood sugar a few hours after a meal when you feel a little hunger because the glucose level in your blood has fallen just below the normal level line. Taking it out of the multiple cycles that occur within your body, I like to simplify it with this reasoning:

After eating, your glucose becomes elevated and insulin drives it back down. It may go to a slightly low level where you sense the "fake hunger syndrome." You're going to get that glucose level back up to the normal line by one of two ways. Either you'll take it in through eating some food, or your body will break down fat tissue to get it transformed into glucose. If you eat that snack, there will be no breaking down of that excess fat you're carrying around. If you don't take those extra calories in through your mouth, your body will provide them through fat breakdown. If you do supply them through some food, the fat stays where it is. What I just explained is not the scientific step-by-step way the body does it, but it is a simple way to understand how you can lose that excess weight. If you eat when you have fake hunger, you're not going to lose any excess weight at that time.

A report in *Nutritional Journal* details how glucose is used in our bodies. The article points out that the sensation of hunger is one of the factors that drives people to overeat, adding additional calories that keep them from losing weight. The article points out that certain foods give a different perception of hunger. You eat them, and you don't have that spike in glucose level nor the big drop that makes you think you need a snack. These foods are similar to the ones you've been encouraged to begin eating on a regular basis—vegetables, fruits, beans, nuts, seeds, and whole grains—while avoiding processed foods and animal products. The higher-fiber foods prevent that sensation of hunger you get during that fake hunger period after meals.

It may take you some time and effort to beat this fake hunger period, but it will be worth it to avoid eating those extra calories just because you think you have low sugar. In step 3, you may have "lower" sugar, but not "low" sugar. Avoid snacks, because most of the time you don't need them.

Weight Loss That Lasts a Lifetime

Once you reach your ideal weight, what do you do differently to ensure that you maintain your ideal weight for the rest of your life? Nothing. Nothing at all. That is the primary benefit of this diet plan. Only 2 to 20 percent of people who have lost weight maintain that loss. That's because most people haven't beaten their addiction for certain foods. They return to their past habits and inevitably regain weight. If you don't abstain and beat the desire, you will fail.

You're different. By following this plan, you'll change your eating habits while you lose weight and continue them for life. You may have a snack now and then if you want, but you will limit any snack to two food types: nuts and fruits. You'll have beaten your desires for the wrong foods. You'll maintain your weight loss.

Now that you know the secrets, act on them. Set your goals. Goals lead to habits, and habits develop into routines. The day will come when what you choose to eat at home or order in a restaurant will become routine. Begin seeing yourself as healthy. Think about it when you first get up and just before you go to bed. Picture yourself trim, with normal blood pressure and normal blood sugar. Think about becoming healthier as you plan what to eat today. Think of what you'll do between meals if you want a snack, what you will drink in its place, what else you can do for the next ten minutes.

If you write down what you're going to do, what you're going to become, you will do it. Set your goals for success in defeating diabetes and write them down. As I've said before, writing down a goal is almost like magic. Get a notebook. Be specific. Write down your goal weight. Write down your menu for each meal for a week. Write down where you're going to exercise each day and what exercise you'll do. Write down when you'll exercise and what clothes you'll wear. Once you believe in setting your goals, you will believe you can change. Believe in it because it can work. I guarantee you will see a difference in what you do.

How Important Is Maintaining Weight Loss in Defeating Diabetes?

The three lifestyle changes—exercise, eating the right foods, and getting to an ideal weight—are intertwined. However, *the most significant factor in defeating diabetes is getting to an ideal weight and maintaining it.*

Let's look at one more study.

An article published in the *American Journal of Medicine* makes the following attention-getting statement about the relationship between being overweight and diabetes: "Some 80% to 90% of persons with type 2 diabetes are overweight." The study further emphasized the other medical problems that occur with diabetics who are overweight. These included an increase in their blood glucose, LDL cholesterol, blood pressure, and heart failure. The study mentioned that weight loss will improve your glucose control as well as your insulin sensitivity. It improves your blood pressure and your cholesterol as well as protects your heart. So any way you look at it, being overweight is bad and losing the excess is excellent.

Then they made a sad, sad statement: "The majority of obese patients regain most of the weight they lose." Why does this happen? Because they didn't lose the desire for certain foods as they lost their excess weight. So when they got to their goal weight, they still had the desire for the bad foods they previously ate, which caused them to gain weight in the first place.

The second reason so many people regain weight after going through the battle of losing it is inactivity. Your odds of keeping your excess weight off are almost nil if you don't continue the exercise routine you developed in losing your weight.

Do what's necessary to not only reach your ideal weight, but to keep it off for life.

Conclusion

Medical research points us to the right path. Remember, you are at a fork in your road of life as a diabetic. Only you can choose which path you're going to take. One can lead to a terrible, disastrous, complicated life, but I encourage you to journey on the road to quality living instead.

You may have recently been diagnosed as diabetic or told you're prediabetic. Or maybe you're afraid you may be diabetic, but you don't want to see your doctor and get that news.

Let me tell you a story about someone I'll call Bill, a diabetic for many years. I had talked to him before about his habits, but he never committed to doing all he could to improve his health. I hope Bill's story will remind you of the dangers of staying on the diabetic road.

Bill was in his late sixties, way overweight, and had been diabetic for many years. I hadn't seen him in over a year when he and his wife came from Georgia to the North Carolina mountains for a long weekend and dropped by our house for a short visit. He got both feet planted on the driveway and stood holding on to the opened car door for a few seconds, smiled, and then moved slowly toward our front door. After we settled into the den, he began telling me about his medical problems, which had developed over the past six months. "My legs are my biggest concern." He pulled up one pants leg to show me how swollen his legs had become.

With my thumb, I gently pressed on the side of his calf. It was like pushing into a thickened sponge. I continued pressing as I watched the end of my thumb sink into the side of his leg. After almost a minute, I told him, "When I remove my thumb, I want you to look at the huge dimple it leaves. It will be the size of a donut hole." I had a slight smile as I looked up at him. "You know, the size of the hole in all those donuts you like to eat."

"I don't eat nearly as many as I used to, Doc. Not since I got started on insulin three years ago." He laughed.

I removed my thumb and the dimple became evident. It sank a good half inch into the soft tissue under the skin. In years past, I had spoken to him on several occasions about his diabetes. Bill had a pattern. He would be energetic about change for a spell but then go right back to his old habits: not watching what he ate, not exercising, regaining his weight. With the new problem of his legs swelling, I realized this meeting could be the last time I might have the chance to motivate him and explain what would happen if he didn't make changes in his lifestyle. My approach was more forceful than in previous conversations.

"Your biggest problem is not your legs. Your biggest problem is your heart."

"Well, that too. My doctor told me it's congestive heart failure."

"Exactly. Your heart is so weak it can't keep your circulation pumping properly throughout your body. Excess fluid is accumulating in your legs. Your heart is failing, and that's what's going to kill you if you don't do something about it. Your diabetes has a lot to do with the health of your heart." I wasn't going to sugarcoat what his future looked like if he didn't change his lifestyle.

"You are on your way out, Bill. Slowly but surely. I can assure you of that. But you can do a lot to extend your time here on earth by many years. We've talked about it before, but you've gotten yourself on a slippery slope. You started out letting yourself get a little overweight, and then you added more and more pounds. And look at where you are now."

"I know." Bill responded. "I've lost fifteen pounds in the past two months. You may not believe me, but I've cut way down on fried foods. And you know what?" I could tell he was about to brag about himself by the way he smiled. "You know how I love biscuits and gravy? Every morning? But now, I only eat them occasionally—"

"Zero," I said, interrupting him. "No more biscuits and gravy. You're at a point in your life where you're going to have to make some major changes."

"But my doctor said I could have them once in a while. He talked to me about not eating them every morning for breakfast, although that has always been my favorite. I don't eat them often, now. Just sometimes on Saturdays." He laughed and slapped me on my shoulder.

"Okay. Let me ask you a question. If you were sitting here talking to someone who smoked, who had a spot on his lung that could be lung cancer, and you told him he had to quit smoking, do you think it would be all right if he said he would quit except smoking one cigarette every Saturday? No, he would need to abstain completely. You must beat the desire for certain foods. Not only foods that harm your diabetes but those that harm your heart. Diabetes plays a huge role in injuring your heart. That's why you're in congestive heart failure right now. You're not going to die from your diabetes; you're going to die from your heart problem.

"It takes about two months to beat the desire for a food addiction, like your biscuits and gravy. That takes abstaining completely. Once the desire begins to fade, I guarantee you, Bill, the day will come when you'll run from those biscuits and gravy because you'll know what harm they'll do to you. And if you will follow my advice, the day will come when you're walking thirty minutes to an hour every day and you'll have become nice and trim."

He looked down at his leg. The donut hole had refilled with fluid and was now as swollen as the rest of his leg. He slid his pants leg back down to his ankle before he looked up at me. "Years ago, when we talked about my diabetes, before I had to start taking insulin, you told me I needed to lose weight. We were talking then about what I needed to do for my diabetes. Now you're saying diabetes affected my heart?"

"Right." I nodded. "When you think 'diabetes,' think 'heart.' It's a double-edged sword, and not many diabetics realize that."

Bill had no idea about the danger diabetes was to his heart. He didn't realize that when diabetics come to the end of their lives, more than 80 percent of the time the finale is a heart attack or stroke. Most diabetics like Bill are fighting the battle of diabetes—checking their blood sugar, pricking their finger multiple times, re-gauging the amount of insulin by the amount of certain sugary foods they eat—but they don't realize the importance of protecting their arteries at the same time. They're fighting only half the fight in the battle of diabetes. Like Bill, all diabetics need to fight the full fight.

I continued. "Do you know anyone who has had a stroke?"

"I sure do. One of my uncles had two of them. The first one left him unable to use his left arm at all, and he walked funny, but he got around real good with a cane."

"What about his second one?"

"It killed him." Bill leaned back on the sofa, shaking his head. "Killed him dead." Bill's Georgia accent said it well.

"Was he a diabetic?"

"Yes, he was. But he didn't take care of himself."

"So he was overweight like you?"

"Oh, he was a lot heavier than me."

Bill's wife decided to chime in. "Bill, he wasn't that much heavier than you."

"Did he have high blood pressure?" I asked.

"He took blood pressure pills for years. As long as I knew him, he had to take a lot of medicine."

I began a sermonette I had preached to him several times in the past. "Bill, after seeing the swelling in your legs, I want to be perfectly straightforward with you. I have known you for many years, and I recall we've talked about what you could be doing to improve your health: what foods to eat, an exercise program, reducing your weight."

"I know, and I really appreciate all the advice you've given me. And you remember I started walking every day."

"That lasted about two weeks each time." His wife chimed in again.

"I don't eat anything like I used to. I've cut down on a lot of what you told me not to eat—"

"You can't just 'cut down,'" I said, interrupting again. "You need to abstain from all the bad foods that affect your arteries. Diabetes harms arteries throughout your body, and you need to do all you can to protect them."

Bill nodded. "A friend was diabetic, and he lost both his legs. I didn't know it was because he was diabetic, though. Are you saying that's why he lost his legs?"

I knew I had his attention at last. "You have congestive heart failure, which means your heart isn't strong enough to pump your blood and fluids around in your body. Your heart muscle is weak because the arteries in your heart aren't letting enough blood through to feed those muscles. Your legs look like water balloons, and that's because your heart is failing. Bill, if you don't change something, this is going to lead to your death.

"You mentioned your uncle had a stroke. That was because the arteries leading to and the arteries within his brain didn't let enough blood into his brain to keep it functioning normally. Am I making sense about how important the blood supply to your heart and brain is? Diabetes makes it all worse."

"I didn't know that—but if you say so." He nodded again.

"Well, I'm saying so, and I'm being blunter with you today because I don't want to lose you. You understand what I'm saying?"

He nodded again, looking more serious.

"Let me give you some things to think about. Did you know you can add years to your life if you'll change your habits to not only improve your diabetes but to also protect your arteries that supply your heart and brain? It's estimated that if you take heart disease and stroke together, 84 percent of people sixty-five or older who have diabetes die from some form of heart disease or a stroke. Eighty-four percent. Remember that number, Bill. That's your destination unless you change the course you're on.

"Anyone who has diabetes needs to do all they can to bring it under control. I'm not saying you'll completely get off your insulin, but many diabetics on insulin do get off it, and some even get off all diabetic medication.

"If someone has diabetes, they're two to four times more likely to die from heart disease than a nondiabetic. Your heart is failing." I paused to let my words sink in. "And you are still way overweight."

I looked directly at him. "Weight loss is a must. Bill, it's do-or-die. Literally. Losing your excess weight not only fights the insulin resistance but also plays a significant role in whipping your heart problem."

I reminded him about how bad high blood pressure was for him. I pointed out that 80 percent of diabetics have high blood pressure and that it adds to the problem with his heart failing. If you have diabetes and high blood pressure, you have more than a twofold risk of dying from your heart problem than someone who has high blood pressure but is not diabetic.

"Bill, when you were here a few years ago, we talked about the importance of exercise. I remember the next day I watched you walking through the neighborhood for over an hour. Remember?"

"Yes. And you know I lost some weight." He started smiling as big as possible.

"That lasted about a week, Bill." His wife was still keeping the story honest. "You didn't walk any after we got back home, not once." She sat with her arms folded.

"Do you exercise any now?" I asked.

"About all the exercise he gets now is when he points the remote at the television," his wife said.

"Here's the deal, Bill. Exercise of any sort, whether you're walking or jogging, swimming, or riding a bike, is one of those things you can control. You either exercise or you don't. Bill, it's up to you. If you don't exercise, your insulin resistance is going to become greater and greater. Being inactive is a huge factor that increases your risk of having problems with your heart.

"Right now, your problem is heart failure. Your next problem could be a blockage of your arteries in your heart causing a heart attack. A couch potato diabetic has a higher risk of having a heart attack than one who exercises. Am I making sense to you?"

"You're scaring me a little bit."

"One, you're way overweight. And two, you don't exercise. You can do something about this, but you must make the decision to do it. You have to want to give the rest of your life more quality than you now have. You have to go beyond the 'want to' aspect to a commitment to do everything we've been discussing. The one question I have is this: Do you think you can do it?"

"Yes, I can. Where do I start?" Bill's jovial voice and smile said it all.

"I would encourage you to make exercise the number one goal you make for yourself today." I looked over at his wife and back to Bill. "She will keep you honest. What do you say?"

"So what's the most important thing I need to do?" Bill asked.

"Losing weight is the most important, but exercise is so significant in weight loss that committing to exercise five to six days a week is the most important thing you can do to convince yourself that you're serious about losing your extra weight."

"Okay. I can at least get started with my walking."

"I know you can do it. So do it."

Bill and I went on to talk about good and bad foods to eat and about how his high cholesterol was connected to both his diabetes and his heart. "Bill, what I'm trying to get across is that you can begin taking some steps you haven't taken in the past, which can reduce your chance of having a heart attack or a stroke and dying earlier than you should."

"You know," he quickly said, "for the first time, I think I'm getting what you're telling me."

Bill drove away that day knowing a lot more about the relationship between diabetes and his heart, and now you know a lot more about steps you can take that will allow you to live a healthier, more active, quality life. I hope Bill's story has been a helpful review of some of the main points we've been covering. I also hope it will act as one of those triggers that will inspire you to take the proper road to defeat diabetes in your life.

I wish you well on your new journey, and I tell you the same as I told Bill: I know you can do it—SO DO IT!

Afterword

If you follow the changes encouraged in this book, you will live extra years. But I want you to think about more than extra years; I want you to think about the quality of every day, every year. Extra years don't count unless quality is associated with those years.

Yet there's more to life than the quality of your years all the way to the end. I want to share what I've learned through some personal experiences as a physician that make me aware of the time *beyond* the end of life. I hope it will help you put diabetes into an even greater perspective.

I have had the opportunity to travel to many areas throughout the world, operating at mission hospitals and providing emergency relief in times of natural disasters. I will never forget an event that made me aware how fleeting this life can be. I was riding in a car down a street only a few days after the 2010 earthquake in Haiti when I saw a car crushed by a concrete slab from a collapsed building. As I looked more closely I saw an arm protruding out of the driver's side. We pulled our car to the side of the street, and I jumped out and ran back to the slab. It was immediately apparent the driver of the crushed car must have escaped, but the lady in the right front seat was only able to lean toward the opened driver's door. She was crushed with only her arm protruding from under the slab.

Then I noticed a bicycle wheel sticking out from under the same slab, just behind the car. I went to my hands and knees and looked under the slab. The man who'd been riding the bicycle was crushed from the waist down, still on the seat. His face and shoulders and arms were all intact, with a plastic water bottle lying just under his outstretched left hand.

The phrase "in the twinkling of an eye" ran through my mind as I looked at these victims. They had both died in just a mere moment of time. Whether we're in great health or have diabetes or high blood pressure or disease of the arteries in our heart, we will all perish someday.

I want to share with you what we tell young doctors Samaritan's Purse sends to the mission field just after they've completed their medical residencies. We explain that we want to support them as well as the hospital where they'll be working, and that their medical expertise will be the platform upon which they'll work in a foreign culture. We want them to be the very best physicians possible to build that platform. From that stage, they will also be able to tell others about the significance of eternity. We remind them that the medical health of their patient is foremost in their hands, but even more significant than a patient's physical health is their spiritual health. One day the physical life will cease, but the spiritual life will last for eternity.

As I conclude this book, I want to share an event that made me more aware of the importance of any individual's spiritual health as well as their physical health.

I was operating in Africa, in a country that didn't have the medical care we enjoy in the United States. The patient's name was Debbie. She was eight years old and had an abdominal mass so large that it made her abdomen protrude. It was easily palpated when she was lying down. In surgery, we found the mass behind her intestine in what is called the retroperitoneal space. That made it inoperable. There was no way to surgically remove the huge tumor. I took a biopsy piece for diagnostic study and closed her abdomen.

I knew the little girl's chances for survival with such a cancer were essentially zero. When I asked the mission doctor where we could send her for chemotherapy, he told me there was no such treatment in the country. I asked what we could do. His reply was that we could do everything possible to keep her comfortable and out of pain, and that we could take better care of her than she could receive anywhere else.

"But," he said, "sometimes the only thing we can do is make certain a patient and their family know about the hope available for eternity. That's the only hope we can give." I was with him as he told Debbie and her parents what we had found. His favorite verse in such situations was John 14:6, when Jesus's disciples asked how they could know the way: "Jesus answered, 'I am the way and the truth and the life. No one comes to the Father except through me.'"

That was a good verse for the family, and it was a good verse to help me contemplate eternity. I decided to begin talking about eternity to my cancer patients back home. I was reminded that anyone who's been given a cancer diagnosis must contemplate what will happen at the end of this life, and from that time forward I always asked patients to whom I'd had to give the diagnosis of cancer if they would like to talk about eternity. Every one of them said yes.

I pointed to the door in my examining room and asked, "If that were the door to heaven and you knocked on it and someone opened it, what could you say that would make them let you in?"

About 80 percent of my patients replied that they hoped they had done more good than bad. Then I told them the verse I learned after operating on Debbie, which let them realize that doing good was not the answer. Jesus was their hope for eternity.

As you finish reading this book about diabetes, my hope is that it will change your life for the good, that it will be a trigger to begin your plan for how you eat, getting to an ideal goal weight, and starting or sustaining your personal exercise program. And last but not least, that this afterword will be a trigger to help you look at eternity differently than you might have before.

I ask you the same question: If you were to stand at the door to heaven and knock, and someone opened it, what could you say that would make them let you in?

My answer is what Jesus said: no one comes to God except through him. And because of that, I have accepted God's Son as my Savior.

It's my desire that you will be able to give the same answer and make the same commitment.

Medical References

American Heart Association

"Cardiovascular Disease & Diabetes." https://www.heart.org/en
/health-topics/diabetes/why-diabetes-matters/cardiovascular
-disease—diabetes. Accessed October 25, 2017.

American Journal of Cardiology

Deedwania PC. Diabetes and vascular disease: common links in the
emerging epidemic of coronary artery disease. 2003 Jan 1; 91 (1):
68–71.

American Journal of Clinical Nutrition

Pan A, Sun Q, Bernstein AM, Schulze MB, Manson JE, Willett WC,
Hu FB. Red meat consumption and risk of type 2 diabetes: 3 cohorts of US adults and an updated meta-analysis. 2011 Oct; 94 (4):
1088–96.

Kaushik M, Mozaffarian D, Spiegelman D, Manson JE, Willett WC,
Hu FB. Long-chain omega-3 fatty acids, fish intake, and the risk of
type 2 diabetes mellitus. 2009 Sep; 90 (3): 613–20.

Halton TL, Willett WC, Liu S, Manson JE, Stampfer MJ, Hu FB.
Potato and French fry consumption and risk of type 2 diabetes in
women. 2006 Feb; 83 (2): 284–90.

Wing RR, Phelan S. Long-term weight loss maintenance. 2005 Jul; 82
(1 Suppl): 222S–225S.

Sabaté J. Nut consumption and body weight. 2003 Sep; 78 (3 Suppl): 647S–650S.

Pereira MA, Jacobs DR Jr, Pins JJ, Raatz SK, Gross MD, Slavin JL, Seaquist ER. Effect of whole grains on insulin sensitivity in overweight hyperinsulinemic adults. 2002 May; 75 (5): 848–55.

Salmerón J, Hu FB, Manson JE, Stampfer MJ, Colditz GA, Rimm EB, Willett WC. Dietary fat intake and risk of type 2 diabetes in women. 2001 Jun; 73 (6): 1019–26.

Meyer KA, Kushi LH, Jacobs DR Jr, Slavin J, Sellers TA, Folsom AR. Carbohydrates, dietary fiber, and incident type 2 diabetes in older women. 2000 Apr; 71 (4): 921–30.

American Journal of Medicine

Norris SL, Zhang X, Avenell A, Gregg E, Bowman B, Serdula M, Brown TJ, Schmid CH, Lau J. Long-term effectiveness of lifestyle and behavioral weight loss interventions in adults with type 2 diabetes: a meta-analysis. 2004 Nov 15; 117 (10): 762–74.

Ascherio A. Epidemiologic studies on dietary fats and coronary heart disease. 2002 Dec 30; (113 Suppl 9B): 9S–12S.

Annals of Internal Medicine

Foster GD, Wyatt HR, Hill JO, Makris AP, Rosenbaum DL, Brill C, Stein RI, Mohammed BS, Miller B, Rader DJ, Zemel B, Wadden TA, Tenhave T, Newcomb CW, Klein S. Weight and metabolic outcomes after 2 years on a low-carbohydrate versus low-fat diet: a randomized trial. 2010 Aug 3; 153 (3): 147–57.

Esposito K, Maiorino MI, Ciotola M, Di Palo C, Scognamiglio P, Gicchino M, Petrizzo M, Saccomanno F, Beneduce F, Ceriello A, Giugliano D. Effects of a Mediterranean-style diet on the need for antihyperglycemic drug therapy in patients with newly diagnosed type 2 diabetes: a randomized trial. 2009 Sep 1; 151 (5): 306–14. Erratum in: Ann Intern Med. 2009 Oct 20; 151 (8): 591.

Orchard TJ, Temprosa M, Goldberg R, Haffner S, Ratner R, Marcovina S, Fowler S; Diabetes Prevention Program Research Group. The effect of metformin and intensive lifestyle intervention on the metabolic syndrome: the Diabetes Prevention Program randomized trial. 2005 Apr 19; 142 (8): 611–9.

Hu FB, Stampfer MJ, Solomon C, Liu S, Colditz GA, Speizer FE, Willett WC, Manson JE. Physical activity and risk for cardiovascular events in diabetic women. 2001 Jan 16; 134 (2): 96–105.

Wei M, Gibbons LW, Kampert JB, Nichaman MZ, Blair SN. Low cardiorespiratory fitness and physical inactivity as predictors of mortality in men with type 2 diabetes. 2000 Apr 18; 132 (8): 605–11.

Archives of Internal Medicine

Sluik D, Buijsse B, Muckelbauer R, Kaaks R, Teucher B, Johnsen NF, Tjønneland A, Overvad K, Ostergaard JN, Amiano P, Ardanaz E, Bendinelli B, Pala V, Tumino R, Ricceri F, Mattiello A, Spijkerman AM, Monninkhof EM, May AM, Franks PW, Nilsson PM, Wennberg P, Rolandsson O, Fagherazzi G, Boutron-Ruault MC, Clavel-Chapelon F, Castaño JM, Gallo V, Boeing H, Nöthlings U. Physical Activity and Mortality in Individuals with Diabetes Mellitus: A Prospective Study and Meta-analysis. 2012 Sep 24; 172 (17): 1285–95.

Look AHEAD Research Group, Wing RR. Long-term effects of a lifestyle intervention on weight and cardiovascular risk factors in individuals with type 2 diabetes mellitus: four-year results of the Look AHEAD trial. 2010 Sep 27; 170 (17): 1566–75.

Fung TT, Schulze M, Manson JE, Willett WC, Hu FB. Dietary patterns, meat intake, and the risk of type 2 diabetes in women. 2004 Nov 8; 164 (20): 2235–40.

Hu FB, Manson JE. Walking: the best medicine for diabetes? 2003 Jun 23; 163 (12): 1397–8.

Albert CM, Gaziano JM, Willett WC, Manson JE. Nut consumption and decreased risk of sudden cardiac death in the Physicians' Health Study. 2002 Jun 24; 162 (12): 1382–7.

Fraser GE, Shavlik DJ. Ten years of life: Is it a matter of choice? 2001 Jul 9; 161 (13): 1645–52.

Fraser GE, Sabaté J, Beeson WL, Strahan TM. A possible protective effect of nut consumption on risk of coronary heart disease. The Adventist Health Study. 1992 Jul; 152 (7): 1416–24.

Biochemical Journal

Barbarroja N, López-Pedrera R, Mayas MD, García-Fuentes E, Garrido-Sánchez L, Macías-González M, El Bekay R, Vidal-Puig A,

Tinahones FJ. The obese healthy paradox: is inflammation the answer? 2010 Aug 15; 430 (1): 141–9.

BMC Endocrine Disorders

Harish K, Dharmalingam M, Himanshu M. Study Protocol: insulin and its role in cancer. 2007 Oct 22; 7:10.

BMJ: British Medical Journal

Stegenga H, Haines A, Jones K, Wilding J; Guideline Development Group. Identification, assessment, and management of overweight and obesity: summary of updated NICE guidance. 2014 Nov 27; 349: g6608.

Floegel A, Pischon T. Low carbohydrate-high protein diets. 2012 Jun 19; 344: e3801. doi: 10.1136/bmj.e3801.

Carter P, Gray LJ, Troughton J, Khunti K, Davies MJ. Fruit and vegetable intake and incidence of type 2 diabetes mellitus: systematic review and meta-analysis. 2010 Aug 18; 341: c4229.

Gillies CL, Abrams KR, Lambert PC, Cooper NJ, Sutton AJ, Hsu RT, Khunti K. Pharmacological and lifestyle interventions to prevent or delay type 2 diabetes in people with impaired glucose tolerance: systematic review and meta-analysis. 2007 Feb 10; 334 (7588): 299.

Wahrenberg H, Hertel K, Leijonhufvud BM, Persson LG, Toft E, Arner P. Use of waist circumference to predict insulin resistance: retrospective study. 2005 Jun 11; 330 (7504): 1363–4.

BMJ Open Diabetes Research & Care

Hamdy O, Mottalib A, Morsi A, El-Sayed N, Goebel-Fabbri A, Arathuzik G, Shahar J, Kirpitch A, Zrebiec J. Long-term effect of intensive lifestyle intervention on cardiovascular risk factors in patients with diabetes in real-world clinical practice: a 5-year longitudinal study. 2017 Jan 4; 5 (1): e000259.

Canadian Journal of Diabetes

Canadian Diabetes Association Clinical Practice Guidelines Expert Committee, Wharton S, Sharma AM, Lau DC. Weight management in diabetes. 2013 Apr; (37 Suppl 1): S82–6.

Centers for Disease Control and Prevention

National Diabetes Statistics Report, 2014. https://www.cdc.gov/diabetes /data/statistics-report/index.html. Accessed October 15, 2018.

Circulation

Jensen MD, Ryan DH, Apovian CM, Ard JD, Comuzzie AG, Donato KA, Hu FB, Hubbard VS, Jakicic JM, Kushner RF, Loria CM, Millen BE, Nonas CA, Pi-Sunyer FX, Stevens J, Stevens VJ, Wadden TA, Wolfe BM, Yanovski SZ, Jordan HS, Kendall KA, Lux LJ, Mentor-Marcel R, Morgan LC, Trisolini MG, Wnek J, Anderson JL, Halperin JL, Albert NM, Bozkurt B, Brindis RG, Curtis LH, DeMets D, Hochman JS, Kovacs RJ, Ohman EM, Pressler SJ, Sellke FW, Shen WK, Smith SC Jr, Tomaselli GF; American College of Cardiology/American Heart Association Task Force on Practice Guidelines; The Obesity Society. 2013 AHA/ACC/TOS guideline for the management of overweight and obesity in adults: a report of the American College of Cardiology/American Heart Association Task Force on Practice Guidelines and The Obesity Society. 2014 Jun 24; 129 (25 Suppl 2): S102–38.

Cornier MA, Després JP, Davis N, Grossniklaus DA, Klein S, Lamarche B, Lopez-Jimenez F, Rao G, St-Onge MP, Towfighi A, Poirier P; American Heart Association Obesity Committee of the Council on Nutrition; Physical Activity and Metabolism; Council on Arteriosclerosis; Thrombosis and Vascular Biology; Council on Cardiovascular Disease in the Young; Council on Cardiovascular Radiology and Intervention; Council on Cardiovascular Nursing, Council on Epidemiology and Prevention; Council on the Kidney in Cardiovascular Disease, and Stroke Council. Assessing adiposity: a scientific statement from the American Heart Association. 2011 Nov 1; 124 (18): 1996–2019.

Ros E, Núñez I, Pérez-Heras A, Serra M, Gilabert R, Casals E, Deulofeu R. A walnut diet improves endothelial function in hypercholesterolemic subjects: a randomized crossover trial. 2004 Apr 6; 109 (13): 1609–14.

Cleveland Clinic Journal of Medicine

Kirwan JP, Sacks J, Nieuwoudt S. The essential role of exercise in the management of type 2 diabetes. 2017 Jul; 84 (7 Suppl 1): S15–S21.

Clinical Edge: "Preventing T2D Through Lifestyle Change Programs." Diabetes Care; ePub 2017 Jul 21; Ely, et al.; August 8, 2017; https:// www.mdedge.com/ccjm/clinical-edge/summary/diabetes /preventing-t2d-through-lifestyle-change-programs. Accessed August 16, 2017.

Cochrane Database of Systematic Reviews

Norris SL, Zhang X, Avenell A, Gregg E, Schmid CH, Lau J. Long-term non-pharmacological weight loss interventions for adults with prediabetes. 2005 Apr 18; (2): CD005270.

Current Diabetes Reports

Lovejoy JC. The impact of nuts on diabetes and diabetes risk. 2005 Oct; 5 (5): 379–84.

Current Molecular Pharmacology

Cao W, Ning J, Yang X, Liu Z. Excess exposure to insulin is the primary cause of insulin resistance and its associated atherosclerosis. 2011 Nov; 4 (3): 154–66.

Diabetes Care

American Diabetes Association. (5) Prevention or delay of type 2 diabetes. 2015 Jan; (38 Suppl): S31–2.

Twig G, Afek A, Derazne E, Tzur D, Cukierman-Yaffe T, Gerstein HC, Tirosh A. Diabetes risk among overweight and obese metabolically healthy young adults. 2014 Nov; 37(11): 2989–95. doi: 10.2337 /dc14-0869.

Wing RR, Lang W, Wadden TA, Safford M, Knowler WC, Bertoni AG, Hill JO, Brancati FL, Peters A, Wagenknecht L; Look AHEAD Research Group. Benefits of modest weight loss in improving cardiovascular risk factors in overweight and obese individuals with type 2 diabetes. 2011 Jul; 34 (7): 1481–6. doi: 10.2337/dc10-2415.

Tonstad S, Butler T, Yan R, Fraser GE. Type of vegetarian diet, body weight, and prevalence of type 2 diabetes. 2009 May; 32 (5): 791–6. doi: 10.2337/dc08-1886.

Djoussé L, Gaziano JM, Buring JE, Lee IM. Egg consumption and risk of type 2 diabetes in men and women. 2009 Feb; 32 (2): 295–300. doi: 10.2337/dc08-1271.

Look AHEAD Research Group, Pi-Sunyer X, Blackburn G, Brancati FL, Bray GA, Bright R, Clark JM, Curtis JM, Espeland MA, Foreyt JP, Graves K, Haffner SM, Harrison B, Hill JO, Horton ES, Jakicic J, Jeffery RW, Johnson KC, Kahn S, Kelley DE, Kitabchi AE, Knowler WC, Lewis CE, Maschak-Carey BJ, Montgomery B, Nathan DM, Patricio J, Peters A, Redmon JB, Reeves RS, Ryan DH, Safford M, Van Dorsten B, Wadden TA, Wagenknecht L, Wesche-Thobaben J, Wing RR, Yanovski SZ. Reduction in weight and cardiovascular disease risk factors in individuals with type 2 diabetes: one-year results of the Look AHEAD trial. 2007 Jun; 30 (6): 1374–83.

Bowker SL, Majumdar SR, Veugelers P, Johnson JA. Increased cancer-related mortality for patients with type 2 diabetes who use sulfonyl-ureas or insulin. 2006 Feb; 29 (2): 254–8.

Ibañez J, Izquierdo M, Argüelles I, Forga L, Larrión JL, García-Unciti M, Idoate F, Gorostiaga EM. Twice-weekly progressive resistance training decreases abdominal fat and improves insulin sensitivity in older men with type 2 diabetes. 2005 Mar; 28 (3): 662–7.

Song Y, Manson JE, Buring JE, Liu S. A prospective study of red meat consumption and type 2 diabetes in middle-aged and elderly women: the women's health study. 2004 Sep; 27 (9): 2108–15.

Sigal RJ, Kenny GP, Wasserman DH, Castaneda-Sceppa C. Physical activity/exercise and type 2 diabetes. 2004 Oct; 27 (10): 2518–39.

Wolf AM, Conaway MR, Crowther JQ, Hazen KY, L Nadler J, Oneida B, Bovbjerg VE; Improving Control with Activity and Nutrition (ICAN) Study. Translating lifestyle intervention to practice in obese patients with type 2 diabetes: Improving Control with Activity and Nutrition (ICAN) study. 2004 Jul; 27 (7): 1570–6.

Church TS, Cheng YJ, Earnest CP, Barlow CE, Gibbons LW, Priest EL, Blair SN. Exercise capacity and body composition as predictors of mortality among men with diabetes. 2004 Jan; 27 (1): 83–8.

Lindström J, Louheranta A, Mannelin M, Rastas M, Salminen V, Eriksson J, Uusitupa M, Tuomilehto J; Finnish Diabetes Prevention Study Group. The Finnish Diabetes Prevention Study (DPS): Lifestyle intervention and 3-year results on diet and physical activity. 2003 Dec; 26 (12): 3230–6.

McAuley KA, Williams SM, Mann JI, Goulding A, Chisholm A, Wilson N, Story G, McLay RT, Harper MJ, Jones IE. Intensive lifestyle changes are necessary to improve insulin sensitivity: a randomized controlled trial. 2002 Mar; 25 (3): 445–52.

Lovejoy JC, Smith SR, Champagne CM, Most MM, Lefevre M, DeLany JP, Denkins YM, Rood JC, Veldhuis J, Bray GA. Effects of diets enriched in saturated (palmitic), monounsaturated (oleic), or trans (elaidic) fatty acids on insulin sensitivity and substrate oxidation in healthy adults. 2002 Aug; 25 (8): 1283–8.

Meyer KA, Kushi LH, Jacobs DR Jr, Folsom AR. Dietary fat and incidence of type 2 diabetes in older Iowa women. 2001 Sep; 24 (9): 1528–35.

Diabetologia

Summers LK, Fielding BA, Bradshaw HA, Ilic V, Beysen C, Clark ML, Moore NR, Frayn KN. Substituting dietary saturated fat with polyunsaturated fat changes abdominal fat distribution and improves insulin sensitivity. 2002 Mar; 45 (3): 369–77.

Hu FB, Van Dam RM, Liu S. Diet and risk of Type II diabetes: the role of types of fat and carbohydrate. 2001 Jul; 44 (7): 805–17.

Eriksson J, Lindström J, Valle T, Aunola S, Hämäläinen H, Ilanne-Parikka P, Keinänen-Kiukaanniemi S, Laakso M, Lauhkonen M, Lehto P, Lehtonen A, Louheranta A, Mannelin M, Martikkala V, Rastas M, Sundvall J, Turpeinen A, Viljanen T, Uusitupa M, Tuomilehto J. Prevention of Type II diabetes in subjects with impaired glucose tolerance: the Diabetes Prevention Study (DPS) in Finland. Study design and 1-year interim report on the feasibility of the lifestyle intervention programme. 1999 Jul; 42 (7): 793–801.

Family Practice News

Bruce Jancin. Fitness Sharply Cut Death in High-BMI Diabetics, October 1, 2008. Publish date: October 1, 2008.

Journal of the American College of Cardiology

Jensen MD, Ryan DH, Apovian CM, Ard JD, Comuzzie AG, Donato KA, Hu FB, Hubbard VS, Jakicic JM, Kushner RF, Loria CM, Millen BE, Nonas CA, Pi-Sunyer FX, Stevens J, Stevens VJ, Wadden TA, Wolfe BM, Yanovski SZ; American College of Cardiology/

American Heart Association Task Force on Practice Guidelines; Obesity Society. 2013 AHA/ACC/TOS guideline for the management of overweight and obesity in adults: a report of the American College of Cardiology/American Heart Association Task Force on Practice Guidelines and The Obesity Society. J Am Coll Cardiol. 2014 Jul 1; 63 (25 Pt B): 2985–3023. Erratum in: J Am Coll Cardiol. 2014 Jul 1; 63 (25 Pt B): 3029–30.

Journal of the American College of Nutrition

Anderson JW, Randles KM, Kendall CW, Jenkins DJ. Carbohydrate and fiber recommendations for individuals with diabetes: a quantitative assessment and meta-analysis of the evidence. 2004 Feb; 23 (1): 5–17.

Journal of the American Dietetic Association

Nettleton JA, Steffen LM, Loehr LR, Rosamond WD, Folsom AR. Incident heart failure is associated with lower whole-grain intake and greater high-fat dairy and egg intake in the Atherosclerosis Risk in Communities (ARIC) study. 2008 Nov; 108 (11): 1881–7.

Journal of Cardiovascular Nursing

Turk MW, Yang K, Hravnak M, Sereika SM, Ewing LJ, Burke LE. Randomized clinical trials of weight loss maintenance: a review. 2009 Jan–Feb; 24 (1): 58–80.

Journal of Clinical Endocrinology and Metabolism

Sung KC, Kim SH. Interrelationship between fatty liver and insulin resistance in the development of type 2 diabetes. 2011 Apr; 96 (4): 1093–7. doi: 10.1210/jc.2010–2190.

Tamura Y, Tanaka Y, Sato F, Choi JB, Watada H, Niwa M, Kinoshita J, Ooka A, Kumashiro N, Igarashi Y, Kyogoku S, Maehara T, Kawasumi M, Hirose T, Kawamori R. Effects of diet and exercise on muscle and liver intracellular lipid contents and insulin sensitivity in type 2 diabetic patients. 2005 Jun; 90 (6): 3191–6.

Journal of Human Hypertension

Han GM, Gonzalez S, DeVries D. Combined effect of hyperuricemia and overweight/obesity on the prevalence of hypertension among

US adults: result from the National Health and Nutrition Examination Survey. 2014 Oct; 28 (10): 579–86.

Journal of Internal Medicine

Trichopoulou A, Psaltopoulou T, Orfanos P, Trichopoulos D. Diet and physical activity in relation to overall mortality amongst adult diabetics in a general population cohort. 2006 Jun; 259 (6): 583–91.

Journal of Nutrition

Neuhouser ML, Schwarz Y, Wang C, Breymeyer K, Coronado G, Wang CY, Noar K, Song X, Lampe JW. A low-glycemic load diet reduces serum C-reactive protein and modestly increases adiponectin in overweight and obese adults. 2012 Feb; 142 (2): 369–74.

Li TY, Brennan AM, Wedick NM, Mantzoros C, Rifai N, Hu FB. Regular consumption of nuts is associated with a lower risk of cardiovascular disease in women with type 2 diabetes. 2009 Jul; 139 (7): 1333–8.

Mukuddem-Petersen J, Oosthuizen W, Jerling JC. A systematic review of the effects of nuts on blood lipid profiles in humans. 2005 Sep; 135 (9): 2082–9.

Tucker KL, Hallfrisch J, Qiao N, Muller D, Andres R, Fleg JL; Baltimore Longitudinal Study of Aging. The combination of high fruit and vegetable and low saturated fat intakes is more protective against mortality in aging men than is either alone: the Baltimore Longitudinal Study of Aging. 2005 Mar; 135 (3): 556–61.

Journal of Physical Activity & Health

Catenacci VA, Odgen L, Phelan S, Thomas JG, Hill J, Wing RR, Wyatt H. Dietary habits and weight maintenance success in high versus low exercisers in the National Weight Control Registry. 2014 Nov; 11 (8): 1540–8.

JAMA: Journal of the American Medical Association

Umpierre D, Ribeiro PA, Kramer CK, Leitão CB, Zucatti AT, Azevedo MJ, Gross JL, Ribeiro JP, Schaan BD. Physical activity advice only or structured exercise training and association with HbA1c levels in type 2 diabetes: a systematic review and meta-analysis. 2011 May 4; 305 (17): 1790–9.

Ingelsson E, Sundström J, Arnlöv J, Zethelius B, Lind L. Insulin resistance and risk of congestive heart failure. 2005 Jul 20; 294 (3): 334–41.

Mokdad AH, Ford ES, Bowman BA, Dietz WH, Vinicor F, Bales VS, Marks JS. Prevalence of obesity, diabetes, and obesity-related health risk factors, 2001. 2003 Jan 1; 289 (1): 76–9.

Stewart KJ. Exercise training and the cardiovascular consequences of type 2 diabetes and hypertension: plausible mechanisms for improving cardiovascular health. 2002 Oct 2; 288 (13): 1622–31.

Pereira MA, Jacobs DR Jr, Van Horn L, Slattery ML, Kartashov AI, Ludwig DS. Dairy consumption, obesity, and the insulin resistance syndrome in young adults: the CARDIA Study. 2002 Apr 24; 287 (16): 2081–9.

Boulé NG, Haddad E, Kenny GP, Wells GA, Sigal RJ. Effects of exercise on glycemic control and body mass in type 2 diabetes mellitus: a meta-analysis of controlled clinical trials. 2001 Sep 12; 286 (10): 1218–27.

Hu FB, Stampfer MJ, Rimm EB, Manson JE, Ascherio A, Colditz GA, Rosner BA, Spiegelman D, Speizer FE, Sacks FM, Hennekens CH, Willett WC. A prospective study of egg consumption and risk of cardiovascular disease in men and women. 1999 Apr 21; 281 (15): 1387–94.

Mayer-Davis EJ, D'Agostino R Jr, Karter AJ, Haffner SM, Rewers MJ, Saad M, Bergman RN. Intensity and amount of physical activity in relation to insulin sensitivity: the Insulin Resistance Atherosclerosis Study. 1998 Mar 4; 279 (9): 669–74.

JAMA Internal Medicine

Pan A, Sun Q, Bernstein AM, Manson JE, Willett WC, Hu FB. Changes in red meat consumption and subsequent risk of type 2 diabetes mellitus: three cohorts of US men and women. 2013 Jul 22; 173 (14): 1328–35.

Lancet

Samuel VT, Petersen KF, Shulman GI. Lipid-induced insulin resistance: unravelling the mechanism. 2010 Jun 26; 375 (9733): 2267–77.

Diabetes Prevention Program Research Group, Knowler WC, Fowler SE, Hamman RF, Christophi CA, Hoffman HJ, Brenneman AT, Brown-Friday JO, Goldberg R, Venditti E, Nathan DM. 10-year follow-up of diabetes incidence and weight loss in the Diabetes Prevention Program Outcomes Study. 2009 Nov 14; 374 (9702): 1677–86.

Imai J, Yamada T, Saito T, Ishigaki Y, Hinokio Y, Kotake H, Oka Y, Katagiri H. Eradication of insulin resistance. 2009 Jul 18; 374 (9685): 264.

Sjöholm A, Nyström T. Endothelial inflammation in insulin resistance. 2005 Feb 12–18; 365 (9459): 610–12.

Massachusetts General Hospital Mind, Mood & Memory

"Anti-inflammatory diet helps lower your Alzheimer's Risk." January 2017, 1.

Medicine and Science in Sports and Exercise

Phelan S, Roberts M, Lang W, Wing RR. Empirical evaluation of physical activity recommendations for weight control in women. 2007 Oct; 3 9 (10): 1832–6.

Kelley DE, Goodpaster BH. Effects of exercise on glucose homeostasis in Type 2 diabetes mellitus. 2001 Jun; 33 (6 Suppl): S495–501; discussion S528–9.

Metabolism

Jenkins DJ, Kendall CW, Popovich DG, Vidgen E, Mehling CC, Vuksan V, Ransom TP, Rao AV, Rosenberg-Zand R, Tariq N, Corey P, Jones PJ, Raeini M, Story JA, Furumoto EJ, Illingworth DR, Pappu AS, Connelly PW. Effect of a very-high-fiber vegetable, fruit, and nut diet on serum lipids and colonic function. 2001 Apr; 50 (4): 494–503.

National Diabetes Information Clearinghouse

"Diabetes Prevention Program (DPP)" NIH Publication No. 09–5099, October 2008.

Nature Medicine

Cai D, Yuan M, Frantz DF, Melendez PA, Hansen L, Lee J, Shoelson SE. Local and systemic insulin resistance resulting from hepatic activation of IKK-beta and NF-kappaB. 2005 Feb; 11 (2): 183–90.

New England Journal of Medicine

Semenkovich CF. Insulin Resistance and a Long, Strange Trip. 2016 Apr 7; 374 (14): 1378–9.

Shulman GI. Ectopic fat in insulin resistance, dyslipidemia, and cardiometabolic disease. 2014 Sep 18; 371 (12): 1131–41.

Hu FB, Willett WC, Li T, Stampfer MJ, Colditz GA, Manson JE. Adiposity as compared with physical activity in predicting mortality among women. 2004 Dec 23; 351 (26): 2694–703.

Knowler WC, Barrett-Connor E, Fowler SE, Hamman RF, Lachin JM, Walker EA, Nathan DM; Diabetes Prevention Program Research Group. Reduction in the incidence of type 2 diabetes with lifestyle intervention or metformin. 2002 Feb 7; 346 (6): 393–403.

Hu FB, Manson JE, Stampfer MJ, Colditz G, Liu S, Solomon CG, Willett WC. Diet, lifestyle, and the risk of type 2 diabetes mellitus in women. 2001 Sep 13; 345 (11): 790–7.

Tuomilehto J, Lindström J, Eriksson JG, Valle TT, Hämäläinen H, Ilanne-Parikka P, Keinänen-Kiukaanniemi S, Laakso M, Louheranta A, Rastas M, Salminen V, Uusitupa M; Finnish Diabetes Prevention Study Group. Prevention of type 2 diabetes mellitus by changes in lifestyle among subjects with impaired glucose tolerance. 2001 May 3; 344 (18): 1343–50.

Chandalia M, Garg A, Lutjohann D, Von Bergmann K, Grundy SM, Brinkley LJ. Beneficial effects of high dietary fiber intake in patients with type 2 diabetes mellitus. 2000 May 11; 342 (19): 1392–8.

Helmrich SP, Ragland DR, Leung RW, Paffenbarger RS Jr. Physical activity and reduced occurrence of non-insulin-dependent diabetes mellitus. 1991 Jul 18; 325 (3): 147–52.

Nutrition Journal

Fuhrman J, Sarter B, Glaser D, Acocella S. Changing perceptions of hunger on a high nutrient density diet. 2010 Nov 7; 9:51.

Nutrition, Metabolism, and Cardiovascular Diseases

Psaltopoulou T, Panagiotakos DB, Pitsavos C, Chrysochoou C, Detopoulou P, Skoumas J, Stefanadis C. Dietary antioxidant capacity is inversely associated with diabetes biomarkers: the ATTICA study. 2011 Aug; 21 (8): 561–7.

Ellsworth JL, Kushi LH, Folsom AR. Frequent nut intake and risk of death from coronary heart disease and all causes in postmenopausal women: the Iowa Women's Health Study. 2001 Dec; 11 (6): 372–7.

Obesity Research

Wyatt HR, Grunwald GK, Mosca CL, Klem ML, Wing RR, Hill JO. Long-term weight loss and breakfast in subjects in the National Weight Control Registry. 2002 Feb; 10 (2): 78–82.

Obesity Reviews

Poobalan AS, Aucott LS, Smith WC, Avenell A, Jung R, Broom J. Long-term weight loss effects on all cause mortality in overweight/ obese populations. 2007 Nov; 8 (6): 503–13.

Obesity (Silver Spring)

Catenacci VA, Pan Z, Thomas JG, Ogden LG, Roberts SA, Wyatt HR, Wing RR, Hill JO. Low/no calorie sweetened beverage consumption in the National Weight Control Registry. 2014 Oct; 22 (10): 2244–51.

American College of Cardiology/American Heart Association Task Force on Practice Guidelines, Obesity Expert Panel, 2013. Expert Panel Report: Guidelines (2013) for the management of overweight and obesity in adults. 2014 Jul; (22 Suppl 2): S41–410.

Peairs AT, Rankin JW. Inflammatory response to a high-fat, low-carbohydrate weight loss diet: effect of antioxidants. 2008 Jul; 16 (7): 1573–8.

Turner-McGrievy GM, Barnard ND, Scialli AR. A two-year randomized weight loss trial comparing a vegan diet to a more moderate low-fat diet. 2007 Sep; 15 (9): 2276–81.

Butryn ML, Phelan S, Hill JO, Wing RR. Consistent self-monitoring of weight: a key component of successful weight loss maintenance. 2007 Dec; 15 (12): 3091–6.

Obstetrics and Gynecology

American College of Obstetricians and Gynecologists Committee on Health Care for Underserved Women. Committee opinion no. 591:

challenges for overweight and obese women. 2014 Mar; 123 (3): 726–30. Erratum in: Obstet Gynecol. 2016 Jan; 127 (1): 166.

Progress in Lipid Research

Risérus U, Willett WC, Hu FB. Dietary fats and prevention of type 2 diabetes. Prog Lipid Res. 2009 Jan; 48 (1): 44–51.

The Free Library

Insulin May Boost Cardiovascular Risk in Type 2 Diabetes Patients. (n.d.) (2014). Retrieved Aug 01 2018 from https://www.thefree library.com/Insulin+May+Boost+Cardiovascular+Risk+in+Type +2+Diabetes+Patients.-a076004492. Accessed October 15, 2018.

The National Weight Control Registry NWCR Facts. http://www.nwcr .ws/research/. Accessed October 15, 2018.

Tufts University Health & Nutrition Letter

"Small steps to health habits," June 2017, 6.

"Don't fear fruits' sugars," June 2017, 2.

"Preventing diabetes saves $$$," June 2017, 2.

"Bone-protective effects of exercise," June 2017, 2.

U.S. National Library of Medicine

Clinical Alert: Diet and Exercise Dramatically Delay Type 2 Diabetes; Diabetes Medication Metformin Also Effective, 08 August 2001. https://www.nlm.nih.gov/databases/alerts/diabetes01.html. Last reviewed: 12 March 2018. Last updated: 12 March 2018. First published: 08 August 2001.

Richard Furman, MD, FACS, spent more than thirty years as a vascular surgeon. The author of *Prescription for Life* and *Your Cholesterol Matters*, Furman is past president of the North Carolina Chapter of the American College of Surgeons, past president of the North Carolina Surgical Society, and a two-term governor of the American College of Surgeons. He is cofounder of World Medical Mission, the medical arm of Samaritan's Purse, and is a member of the board of Samaritan's Purse. He lives in Boone, North Carolina. For more information, please visit www.prescription forlifeplan.com.

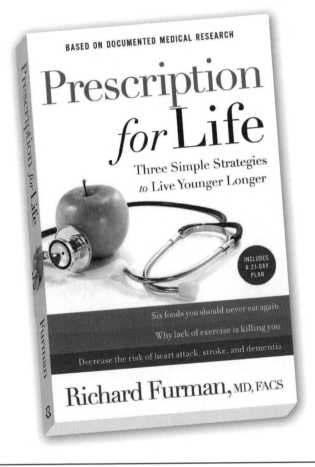
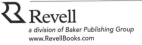

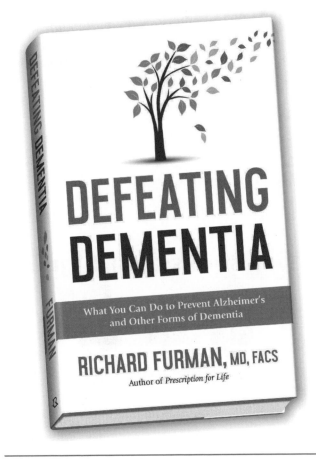

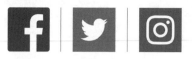
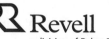